Becoming a Good Doctor:

The Place of Virtue and Character in Medical Ethics

James F. Drane

Sheed & Ward

The Catholic Health Association OF THE UNITED STATES **CHA**

Sheed & Ward™ is a service of National Catholic Reporter Publishing Company, Inc.

Library of Congress Catalog Card Number: 88-61721

ISBN: 1-55612-209-8

Published by: Sheed & Ward
               115 E. Armour Blvd. P.O. Box 419492
               Kansas City, MO 64141-6492

To order, call: (800) 333-7373

Contents

In memory of
Joseph DeFrees

Inventor—Industrialist—Humanist

He used the fruits of his technical
genius to make his world a little better.

Acknowledgments

This book was made possible by the support and encouragement of the Board of Directors of the DeFrees Foundation: Miss Ann DeFrees, Mr. Charles DeFrees, Mrs. June DeFrees Heelan, Mr. Harold Johnson, and Mrs. Barbara DeFrees.

Melissa Curry read my awful handwriting and got the book into typewritten form. Andy Lawlor transcribed the material into an acceptable software system. Prof. Elsie Deal, with care and attention beyond professional standards, edited the text and did the index.

Foreword

The Spanish philosopher Miguel de Unamuno, in the middle of some of his most rigorous philosophical works, would start a conversation with the reader. The person of Unamuno, and not just his mind, was always present in what he wrote, and he engaged the person of the reader directly to ask for an opinion or to solicit a response. This sort of thing does not happen in our culture. The only place one finds personal notes in American books is in a foreword, and so I will take advantage of this space to talk a little about myself and the persons to whom I am indebted for this book.

Twenty-five years ago, I studied philosophy at the University of Madrid with Jose Luis Aranguren. This was not my first experience with European education. Ten years before that I had studied theology at the Gregorian University of Rome. Moral theology then was almost a medical ethics course because so many of the cases illustrating ethical principles came from medicine. Later on in Spain, Aranguren showed me how to rethink my Catholic tradition without abandoning its basic insights. Character and virtue considerations remained central to the ethical enterprise, but these categories were given a new grounding and reexamined in light of contemporary thinkers. It is around these same categories that this book on medical ethics centers.

Jose Luis Aranguren was then, and remains today, the dominant figure in Spanish ethics. He was ahead of his time in interests and concerns and was an engaged rather than simply an armchair thinker. He knew contemporary European philosophy as well as the English and American Analytic tradition. He integrated insights from these other traditions into his own work, without abandoning the Mediterranean tradition where character and virtue considerations were basic. The importance of problem solving was neither ignored nor denied, but ethics was first a matter of the kind of person one came to be by grappling with life. The first part of this book reflects Aranguren's thought and argues for his same basic orientation in ethics.

Studying in Europe twenty-five years ago was different. There was a strong personal dimension to the education I received which one finds only rarely in American graduate schools. Doing graduate study in Spain has more the flavor of becoming a disciple than fulfilling graduate requirements. Dissertations are pretty much the same in both cultures, but what I came away with after finishing my thesis was a friendship with my professor which will last until we die. He had many students, but I felt that he treated me in a special way. I accompanied him on lectures out of town, ate often at his home, became close to all his children, and even went to parties and social occasions with him. The human personal was at the center of Jose Luis Aranguren's ethics, and there was a strong personal dimension to the whole educational experience he provided. This personal dimension is what I've tried to re-introduce into modern American medical ethics.

The most interesting of the social affairs I attended with my professor was an old fashioned European Tertulia (party) which took place every Thursday evening in a Madrid restaurant, where ten to twelve of Spain's outstanding intellectuals met to eat and to talk and to have a good time. The meal lasted for hours, and besides being a pleasant experience, it provided a place for poets, philosophers, novelists, artists, historians, and linguists to talk among themselves and to argue about the issues of the day. Just being at those meals was an education. Five or six hours there went by faster than any class or graduate seminar.

One of the members of this group was the former rector (president) of the University of Madrid, who, unlike typical administrators here, was a widely recognized and much published man of letters. Indeed, Pedro Lain was then and has remained something of a patriarch of Spanish letters. He is a physician, historian, philosopher, literary critic, and well-known essayist. At that time, he had already been elected to the Academy of the Language and the Academy of History and had just been selected to enter the Academy of Medicine. The *Academia*, in Mediterranean countries, is the scholastic version of the Hall of Fame. I can't remember whether Pedro gave me an invitation to the ceremony of induction or whether I accompanied Jose Luis, but I remember the occasion well. Pedro held center stage, adorned like Solomon in the priestly robes of academic life, and surrounded on all sides by fellow academicians, similarly adorned. We sat outside what looked to me like a communion rail as Pedro delivered his induction lecture: "The doctor-patient relationship in the Middle Ages." As I sat there, I remember thinking to myself, "My Lord, who is interested in such a topic, and why would anyone spend time researching and writing about it?"

As it turned out, I came to understand why this was a topic of interest and, in fact, came to be very interested in it myself. A long standing involvement with ethics, joined to an invitation to study at the Menninger School of Psychiatry, got me back in touch with the medical dilemmas which were so much a part of my early theological education. One thing led to another, and in 1985, I went back to Spain to see my friends Pedro Lain and Jose Luis Aranguren and to start working with Pedro on this book. What I first thought would be of interest to no one, I later wound up thinking and writing about.

My relationship with Pedro Lain is similar to the one I have with Jose Luis. Pedro took the same personal interest in me and was always available when I needed help. Many times I was a guest in Pedro's home, spent some special times with his wife, Milagro, learning about the Spanish Civil War, got to know their children and grandchildren and many of their personal friends. Again, I know Pedro has had many students and disciples, but he made me feel special, and I am most indebted, to him for the book.

At the Universidad Pontifica de Comillas (in Madrid) last year, I participated in a seminar which included physicians, scientists, lawyers, philosophers and theologians from around the country. We met every other Saturday for some months. Each participant read a paper and took part in a half day dialogue about it with the other participants. Pedro Lain read a paper ahead of me on doctor-patient friendship, relating the requirements of the ancient virtue of friendship to modern problems like *in vitro* fertilization and genetic engineering. It was like *déja vu*, but this time the questions I had twenty-five years ago about the relevance of his ideas were more than answered. I saw the relationship between those traditional, historical categories and modern medical problems; how that ancient tradition could be made new and relevant to today's concerns.

In my own paper for the seminar, I talked about American style medical ethics; its historical tradition, methodology, categories and objectives. My role at the seminar, I felt, was that of a bridge: bringing our American experience in practical problem solving to Spain where all the most pressing problems are on the ground, but almost everything remains to be done in developing practical methods and structures for finding concrete solutions. I spent time in Spain (during 1987) teaching the first American style bioethics course in the medical school at the University of Madrid. I also traveled around the country trying to get medical ethics started at other medical schools and medical centers. The bridge, however, goes both ways.

This book is an attempt to bring back to the attention of my American colleagues the ideas and orientations of my Spanish friends. No one philosophical tradition or methodology or set of concepts is ever adequate to all the complexities of a reality which needs to be understood. A broad eclectic approach is our best bet for adequacy. Narrow dogmatic methodologies are as obfuscating and unproductive in medical ethics as they are in theology or any other discipline.

And yet the majority of American medical ethicists practice on only one small section of ethical turf. Focused mainly on dilemmas and quandaries, American ethicists work at finding rules and procedures for getting out of a bind. American clinical ethicists tend to be a professional's ally as doctors struggle to make the right choice in this or that particular conflict situation. But this style of ethics really only helps the physician in a tiny area of his or her overall activity. Doctoring is through and through an ethical enterprise. Certainly, doctors need help with decision making in hard cases, but the thousands of other non-conflictual medical acts also have ethical dimensions, and these need to be attended to in medical ethics.

Because modern medical practice has more and more problem areas, guidelines and procedural strategies for decision making in these areas are more and more important. It makes good sense for a profession to grapple with the problem areas of its practice. But not all medical practice is problematic or conflicted. For certain problems, a technically correct procedure or a rule of thumb might suffice. But for other aspects of life what is needed is not a strategy or a rule but rather a style of life, or way of being that fits or is appropriate. Like everyone else, doctors shape the ethical narrative of their lives by the ways they do ordinary things over and over again.

An ethics for the other aspects of life is expressed more commonly in narratives and stories. James Gustafson is another friend and teacher to whom I am indebted, and he tells a story which makes this point.

In the mid-1950's on a hot summer night, a colleague and I had worked past midnight on a report marking the termination of a brief but intensive interdisciplinary study. We left our workroom in a midtown Manhattan hotel to go to the bar for some refreshment. Near us was seated a rather drunken young soldier, who proceeded to order another drink. He paid for it with a twenty dollar bill, but my observing colleague noticed that the bartender gave him change for a five. My colleague insisted that the soldier receive the rest of his change. The bartender protested that the soldier had given him a five, and not a twenty dollar bill. An argument ensued and, finally, the bartender gave the soldier fifteen dollars, asserting that he was doing it only to keep peace in the establishment.

The soldier's inebriation progressed to the point where it was clear that he would soon "pass out." Certainly he was rapidly losing control of his speech and his muscles. My colleague talked to him as best one could in these circumstances and finally took the soldier's wallet from his pocket. There was identification indicating that the young man lived at a Long Island address. We took ten dollars from the wallet, and my colleague wrote a note indicating that we had done so, that we were putting him in a cab and giving the cab driver the ten dollars to take him home. He also gave our names and professions and the telephone number of the hotel in which we were quartered by the corporation for whom we were doing the study. Thus the soldier or his family could make contact with us if they desired any further explanation.

We more or less dragged the soldier onto Lexington Avenue, where we hailed a taxi. My colleague gave the driver the ten dollar bill and the address. He also took the driver's name and license number and indicated that we had the young man's name and address. Thus the driver knew that it would be possible to check out whether the drunken soldier had been delivered home. My colleague also informed the driver that we knew how much money was left in the wallet.

When the taxi drove off, we returned to the bar.*

From this story something can be seen about ethics which does not fit into the typical American language categories of rights and cost-benefit analysis. Ethics is also about excellence, and about style, and about the character of a person who sees what is wrong and tries to make things right. No one would deny that Jim Gustafson's friend acted morally, and yet the morality of his act is hardly understandable in terms of rules or rights or principles of utility. More than likely, the actor in this story formulated his intervention without referring to any of the standards used in contemporary medical ethics. His action was the expression of a certain style of life: a well formed character. What he did was carried out with ease because it was "natural" for him. Obviously, what he did was moral, but its morality goes beyond what rules require or rights can claim. This idea of morality is what the European tradition emphasizes, and it deserves a place in American medical ethics.

The Gustafson story has nothing to do with caring for sick people, but certain generalizations can be drawn from it which apply to medical ethics. We see, for example, how ethics emerges out of a relationship of one person to another. In the first part of this book, the relationship between doctor and patient will be the ground and starting point of a medical ethics which looks to just such examples of virtuous behavior as goals for medical practitioners.

*James M. Gustafson, *Can Ethics Be Christian*. Chicago, University of Chicago Press, 1985. Chapter 1.

Doctors are related to patients in a special way because they profess to be helpers and therefore assume obligations to people who need them. Dependency and a promise to help give relationships an obligatory note that certain character types respond to without much thought to rules and rights. Something of the way in which Jim's friend responded to the helpless drunk marks the way a good doctor responds to persons who are ill.

Some aspects of the doctor-patient relationship and the relationship of Jim's friend and the soldier are fixed and determined. Limitations on action are built in. Yet, at the same time, relationships are full of openings possibilities. The professional is limited by who he or she is; the patient is similarly limited. Yet there are many possibilities within these limits for possible moral actions: good, bad, indifferent, excellent. Both the professional self and the other can be changed by what is decided upon. Excellence in action can change both parties. How one person uses his powers, whether speech, or capacity for friendship, or courage, or diagnostic and therapeutic capabilities, can make both the person of the actor and the person acted upon different and better persons.

How a professional person will act in a relationship depends upon many factors, but images of who he or she wants to be, models of how to act, will have an influence on what actually occurs. Ethics has to do with images, models and ideals that influence character and virtue. These concepts and categories explain better than rules and rights the kind of morality one sees illustrated in this story and in countless unrecorded stories about doctor and patient interactions.

The discipline called ethics attempts to make intelligible experiences of human persons in relationships. To do so, some framework and categories have to be employed. My project of acting as a bridge between Spanish and American ethicists is actually an attempt to join Northern European Protestant categories with a Southern European Catholic framework. The Protestant model centers around duties and rights and formal standards of right and wrong. The other centers on character, virtue and styles of being a good person. Modern medical ethics, in my opinion, needs both. Trying to squeeze experiences like the one recorded in the Gustafson story into a Northern European framework does not do them justice.

No doubt, rules could be teased out of the story and it could be argued that Jim's friend was applying principles and defending rights or weighing consequences. But these categories are not adequate to the experience. There are no rules telling him what he should do in that situation, and none that can tell doctors what to do in many situations they face. And no rule could be found that would require a person to take the subtle and delicate steps to achieve that final excellent result. Doing the excellent thing was a matter of intuiting what was appropriate by a person who had developed a certain way of being; an ethical style of life. Not a great deal of reflection or calculation was required because the actions were natural: habits of character formed by many previous experiences and sustained by moral beliefs, images and ideals. The story illustrates better than any argument that character in many situations is more important than methodology of moral reasoning, rules, principles, rights and the like.

Many a contact between doctor and patient has points of similarity with Jim's story: the relationship, the dependency, the mutuality, the sense of obligation, a naturalness in going beyond what is ordinarily required, the making of oneself and the other by the quality of the intervention. There is a certain *virtuosity* in the action of good doctors which evokes our admiration just as surely as there are falls from goodness which enrage patients and send them looking for legal remedies. This book makes an argument for such personal qualities. The project is a modest one: to raise the question, to open the door, to initiate the discourse in this older Catholic tradition for thinking about modern medical moral experience.

Introduction

Medicine And Medical Ethics Today

In the opening essay of *The Man Who Mistook His Wife for a Hat*, Oliver Sacks tells the fascinating story of a person suffering from agnosia.[1] Dr. P. (the patient) was a distinguished musician, singer and teacher of music in Berlin. It was in relating to his students that certain strange problems were first observed. Suddenly, he could not recognize certain young people, even ones he knew well. Besides not being able to identify people he often mistook objects like parking meters and water hydrants for young children. At the end of one of his sessions with Dr. Sacks, Dr. P started looking around for his hat. He reached out toward his wife's head, and tried to put it on his own.

Agnosia is the psychiatric term for the loss of ability to recognize familiar objects. Dr. P.'s particular illness made him unable to recognize persons. The most personal features of a face he saw in bits and pieces, and as partial shapes. Indeed, he retained a highly abstract and sophisticated cognitive capability, but one which did not include recognizing features. Since human beings were seen only as abstract shapes and categories, an indifference to them followed. Although it seems incredible, Dr. P. got along quite well despite his dreadful disability and was able to work to the very end of his life. He did not suffer from what we would assume to be a terrible loss, and as far as he was concerned, he was getting along quite well. He would have responded positively to any inquiry about the quality of his life.

1

Amusing and yet tragic, Dr. P.'s case provides us with a metaphor for modern medicine and even for modern medical ethics. In our highly technical and scientific medicine, persons are also in danger of being lost: becoming a cluster of abstract signs, symptoms, separate parts and mechanical functions. Like Dr. P., medicine has refined its abstract categorizations of bodies, but has lost contact with the personal features of patients. Like him, modern medicine functions, but in a diminished and depersonalized world. The modern medical practitioner can see very clearly separate parts and their mechanical interactions, but frequently he or she misses the face of the person being treated. The mechanical and the abstract are important; indeed they are the keys to modern medicine's advances. But if after perfecting perception in these areas, personal dimensions are ignored, then medicine, like Dr. P., has become ill.

Everyone familiar with the big, modern hospital knows doctors who consistently fail to recognize the faces of their patients. And, in an odd reversal of roles, patients, not medical professionals, are the first to diagnose this disorder. People with little or no medical sophistication notice that there is something wrong with many doctors.

What is true of medical professionals is true to some extent even of medical ethics, which is also fascinated with abstractions: rules and rights, principles and codes, metaethical theories and computerized schemata for ethical analysis. If doctors can suffer from agnosia, so, too, can ethicists. Calling what one does a literate discipline is not a vaccination against this disease. The object of ethics, not unlike the object of medicine, can become an It, farther and farther removed from the realm of Thou. Oddly enough, there is a certain bliss, or at least an indifference, that accompanies loss of the personal. The Dr. P. story is a parable for much of what happens today in and around medicine.

Even without knowing it, ethicists easily slip into a belief that the good is synonymous with abstract definitions, and doctors slip into practices focused only on numbers, printouts and lab reports. The whole world of human persons, as well as the special respect which persons are owed, can disappear from day to day activities and the meaning of doing good is collapsed into doing things efficiently. Any and every professional is vulnerable to losing touch with the personal, but when this happens in medicine, the loss creates a distortion. Medical ethics courses, one might think, would try to keep this from happening, but even medical ethics can become impersonal.

A report, published in the *New England Journal of Medicine* by a distinguished group of medical ethics educators, reflects this focus on techniques for problem solving, and the objective aspects of the ethical enterprise:

> We believe that the basic medical ethics curriculum should be centered on the kinds of moral problems that physicians encounter most frequently in practice, rather than on sensational cases of the type that occur only rarely. The curriculum should address several different kinds of learning: the clarification of central concepts (e.g., the patient's competence to consent to or refuse treatment); the understanding of important decision-making procedures (e.g., how to determine when it is morally justified to treat an unwilling patient); the ability to apply concepts and decision-making procedures to actual cases; and the acquisition of certain interactional skills (e.g., the ability to discuss with a terminally ill patient his or her wishes about being placed on Do Not Resuscitate status).[2]

Even talking to patients has become a matter of learning objective skills. These educators set objectives for teaching medical ethics to medical students and take the position that attention to a young doctor's personal traits or character is out of place in a medical ethics curriculum:

> Before presenting our recommendation for a basic curriculum, we want to make explicit certain beliefs we hold about the teaching of medical ethics. First of all, we believe that the basic moral character of medical students has been formed by the time they enter medical school. A medical ethics curriculum is designed not to improve the moral character of future physicians, but to provide those of sound moral character with the intellectual tools and inter-

actional skills to give that moral character its best behavioral expression.[3]

This proposal assumes that moral character is important, but holds
that it has no place in ethics courses. Careful selection of candidates, the
educators think, is all that is needed to keep up a certain level of per-
sonalism and moral rectitude among doctors. This strategy, however,
turns out to be problematic for many reasons. Both ethics and character
development are quite universally ignored throughout the educational
system in America. What are the minimal standards of good character
already assumed to be present in the young doctors? And what about the
widely recognized depersonalizing influences on character of medical
education itself? How may these influences be offset? If personal
character has a place in medical ethics, then someone at some time
during training should at least address this issue. But is there any practical and effective way to do so? Much of what has been written about
medical ethics in the past was concerned almost exclusively with personal character, and yet this historical material now seems hopelessly
dated.

Rather than trying to answer all of the above questions, I hope only to
call attention to the personal or character dimensions of doctoring and to
initiate some thinking about these topics. My assumption is that a ven-
erable tradition in ethics that focuses on persons, virtue and character,
has something to say to both younger and older practitioners of medicine
today, and therefore should have a place in modern medical ethics. I will
try to make this point by telling a story of my own.

Before settling down in Madrid to begin work on this book, I stopped
in Paris to visit some old haunts from student days, and to inquire about
the state of medical ethics in the nation of Descartes and rationalism.
Since I had no contacts or letters of introduction, I simply stopped at the
Hotel Dieu one morning and asked to speak to the doctor in charge of the
Neo-natology unit. A young physician appeared who happened to be interested in ethics and we spent quite a while talking in his office. At the
end of the conversation, he gave me the name of a Dr. Alexandre
Minkowski, whom he said was very involved with the national ethics

committee recently formed in France to address problems raised by medical technology. So, the next day I set out to talk to him.

Alexandre Minkowski, it turned out, was a man in his early 70s, large by French standards, robust, Harvard educated, and Jewish. He had just written a book, his seventh, entitled *L'Impertinent (The Impertinent One)*.[4] He thought of himself as being very much influenced by his American education and interpreted this influence primarily in terms of saying exactly what he thought, to whomever, without worrying about being polite. Dr. Minkowski thought of himself as a free-thinker, and although politically Left, he admired the virtues of classic liberalism. It turned out that, contrary to what my first doctor had thought, he was not a member of the ethics committee. In fact, he showed me the pages of his book which ridiculed the prestigious National Ethics Committee and its deliberations. The idea of the state committee made up of distinguished persons, developing rules and guidelines for doctors, he thought, was ridiculous. Listening to him rant about the National Committee, one would think that he was a total and radical relativist; convinced that no one could tell anyone else what to do. At least, that was the position he espoused in our conversation, and the one he continued to defend, even in the face of my objections about Dr. Mengele and the terrible harm this one pathetic physician had done by following his personal convictions alone.

My first impression of the impertinent Dr. Minkowski, however, was not quite accurate. What he actually believed in, I came to understand, was a very traditional medical ethics of character and virtue. It was his belief that the state committee and its rules were unnecessary because doctors with experience already know what is the right thing to do, even in difficult cases. When, in our long conversation, I pressed him about what he meant by experience, it turned out to be more like proven virtue. Built into Dr. Minkowski's approach to medical ethics was an assumption that ethics is a matter of decent (virtuous) doctors doing what they know to be best for their patients. Minkowski, for all his radical posturing and claims of impertinence, was actually an old-fashioned, ethical doctor with largely traditional ideas about medicine and medical ethics.

He assumed, as the medical educator did, either that only persons of good moral character become doctors or that moral character somehow develops through education, or experience, or both.

What Dr. Minkowski did not say explicitly, was that state promoted medical ethics is inadequate because it is too tied to rules and regulations. Minkowski thought he was opposed to medical ethics, but what he opposed was a type of medical ethics which does not consider personal virtue and a doctor's character. He was reacting with ridicule to an account of ethics in medicine which tries to make rules bear the whole weight of the moral perplexities facing today's medicine.

Dr. Minkowski's criticisms of the rules and regulations of the French National Ethics Committee find a subtler and more reasoned articulation in the works of Harry Beecher at the very beginning of the modern era of bioethics.[5] He argued that ethical rules and regulations are likely to do more harm than good, and ultimately will never curb the unscrupulous practitioner. What Beecher proposed, in contrast to the rules and regulations of the Nuremburg Code, was a re-emphasis on traditional virtue ethics and the cultivation of medical virtues in young physicians. He called for a combined emphasis of sound, scientific methodology and sound character training for those who would practice either clinical or experimental medicine. His solution to the dangers of immorality associated with powerful new medical science was a virtuous doctor or researcher, and he listed the virtues he felt were most important: compassion, responsibility, conscientiousness and intelligence. Beecher did not even mention patients' rights. In fact, he was worried about talk of informed consent for either patients or research subjects, feeling that such a requirement would cripple research into mental illness. Beecher's work was important because it focused attention on the complex ethical issues emerging in contemporary medicine. He has been rightly criticized, however, for an exclusive reliance on virtue as the solution.

From the time of Hippocrates, medical codes have appealed for both rules and virtue. Patients were expected to trust their physicians and to follow their advice because doctors were persons of excellent character. Superior personal moral development was considered to be more important than following rules and regulations. Historically, rules and codes were important, but by themselves inadequate to the complexities of medicine. Doctors have always insisted that many medical situations do not permit the luxury of objective analysis and discriminating rule application. Consequently, throughout history, one finds a certain discomfort with rules and codes, especially if they are presumed to bear the whole weight of right and wrong. Medical ethics is not a very popular subject today with doctors. An old discomfort with ethics understood primarily in terms of objective rules and norms, is still alive and well among contemporary practitioners.

Some of this discomfort can be understood, if not totally excused, by looking at developments in medical ethics over the last twenty-five years. With few exceptions, medical ethicists have not been doctors but philosophers, the majority of whom were trained in American universities where linguistic schools of thought held sway. Consequently, the whole medical ethics enterprise has been conceived in terms of logic, principles, patients' rights, and procedures to achieve equality in doctor-patient relationships. What has come to be called medical ethics is the application of an abstract, analytical style of doing ethics to cases generated by medical practice.

An interest on the part of moral philosophers in medicine meant only a new set of examples to which their standard assumptions about ethics were applied. Deontologists and Consequentialists developed arguments for their basic principles (autonomy or utility), and applied these principles to medical quandaries in order to arrive at practical rules. Procedures were developed to bring some order to the bewildering complexities of clinical cases, and then rules were applied to indicate the direction of a defensible course of action. The development of procedural schemata and abstract conceptual categories made it possible to find concrete solutions in tough decision-making situations, and this relieved the moral "dis-ease" of medical practitioners.

Expert practitioners of the new American medical ethics were able to shift their conceptual apparatus without much difficulty from medicine to other professions.[6] Centers of research originally organized for medical ethics developed into centers for the study of ethics in business, government, law and journalism. The shift was easy because the same categories and concepts used for medical problems were simply applied to other professional areas.

The very ease of this shift says something important about American style medical ethics. No one can deny that the heavily logical and practical approach brought clarifications and coherence to the consideration of ethical quandaries in medicine. No one disputes the fact that there is a role in any adequately conceived ethics for logical analysis, principles, rules and procedures. But medicine is different from other professions, and it is this difference which is not reflected in a way of doing ethics which focuses exclusively on objective categories. It was precisely because what is unique to medicine was left out of consideration that this approach could so easily be transferred to other professions.

Case ethics, for example, is important because medicine is always about cases, but there is no place in objective case analysis for considerations of that moral commitment which characterizes the best physicians. The ordinary medical practitioner's moral attitudes are also left out of consideration. The doctor's way of being is given no place in a method designed primarily to resolve conflicts by seeing things in strictly impersonal categories. Perhaps it is the sense that so much of what goes on in medicine is left unarticulated in modern medical ethics that makes physicians like Alexandre Minkowski feel dissatisfied and suspicious of the whole medical ethics enterprise.

Minkowski would be hard for many people to take, but there is no denying that he is a doctor to the very core of his being. The rules of the Ethics Committee, he felt, were ridiculous because they did not reflect the heart, skill, experience and character which he brought to each and every difficult case. Minkowski thought of himself as impertinent and radical, but actually he stood for a traditional approach to ethics. It was moral character that he referred to again and again in terms like, "humanity," "experience" and "personal feelings," and he felt that these were missing in the rule making of the National Committee. Minkowski has the kind of mind that can quickly perceive the insufficiency of national rules and norms for medical practice. But his criticism and ridicule are too facile.

The easiest criticism, even of the most humane objective standard, is to say that it cannot be universally applied in every situation. Such a criticism is superficial and beside the point. Human diversity is too obvious to require proof, but it is also true that human actions have not just a host of unique human characteristics, but commonalities as well, which provide a basis for generalization in the form of rules or standards. Multi-national commissions have worked out agreed upon standards of right and wrong, valid for professionals in very different cultures, e.g., international medical codes. The European community, for example, is made up of cultures which differ in language, religion and political structure, and yet they have agreed upon standards of ethical practice in medicine.[7]

Minkowski's ridicule of norms and rules of conduct also suffers from a lack of critical attention to a virtue-based medical ethics, which he merely assumes will produce the right kind of conduct. There are thinkers at the opposite end of the spectrum who ridicule Minkowski's assumptions that virtue, experience and character will provide solutions to the real problems facing modern medicine.[8] In fact, for medical ethicists like Robert M. Veatch, doctors like Minkowski are dangerous precisely because of their convictions of righteousness. Because they think they know what is right, they suffer from hubris and other forms of blindness, which keep them from seeing and considering the very different value framework of patients. Therefore, they tend more frequently to do the wrong thing than the right. This is a serious objection.

Minkowski is vulnerable to this criticism because he refuses to spell out any objective standards which inform his "experienced and humane treatment of patients." His could be called a naked theory of virtue; virtue understood solely as an experienced, humanistic disposition, an inclination to act in the right way. A radical deontologist like Veatch relies on rules and objective standards of conduct rather than naked physician virtue, and actually goes so far as to say that virtue and character development is dangerous. At face value, this opposite position is itself ridiculous, but a point is being made that is worth taking into account. Minkowski is a humanistic person who enjoys a good professional reputation and yet, for just that reason, his ethical decisions in the complex medical setting would tend to escape public monitoring. Put another way, Minkowski is not sufficiently attentive to the problems created by his own original sin. Even good, decent people can do wrong things even as their self-righteousness and their good public reputation prevent them from recognizing the wrongs. On several celebrated occasions, for example, researchers with just such personal qualities, did some terrible things to helpless, innocent people.[9]

A middle position between the two extremes recognizes, with Minkowski, the importance of character formation and moral virtue in medical practice. But it recognizes too, that any talk of virtue and character needs some type of objective grounding. Talk of virtue and character reduced to pure dispositions is a distortion. The goal of a middle position is the development of a concept of medical character and medical virtue which makes good sense, can influence conduct appropriate to the role of a good doctor, and has a philosophical foundation which gives coherence and solidity to its virtue and character claims. The cultivation of character and virtue once was the meaning of ethics, and retains importance today for groups as diverse as Catholic Moral Theologians and Secular Humanists. Developing a case for the place of virtue and character in modern medical ethics will be the objective of the pages which follow.[10]

Human beings can never be understood in an exhaustive or final way, but we can know something about being human and correspondingly, know that certain conduct is right because it respects, promotes, and is owed to humans. Correspondingly, we can know something about illness, the needs of persons who are ill and the history of the profession which stops to help ill people. Certainly, our understanding is limited, and certainly, there are complications introduced by cultural variations, but there is also trans-cultural agreement about what constitutes both human good and good medical practice. Certain conduct in medicine is recognized as right, and respected among radical feminists, Orthodox

Jews, primitive tribesmen, and the partly secular, residually Christian doctors practicing in any American hospital. Traditional ethics education in medicine was concerned with developing the character of young doctors so they would act habitually in the right way. We will look at this tradition and try to restore its place in medical ethics by bringing it up to date.

Notes

1. Oliver Sacks, *The Man Who Mistook His Wife for a Hat* (New York: Summit Books), 1985.

2. Charles M. Culver, M.D., Ph.D., et al, "Basic Curricular Goals in Medical Ethics," *New England Journal of Medicine*, Jan. 24, 1985, vol. 312, no. 4, p. 253.

3. Ibid., p. 253.

4. Alexandre Minkowski, *L'Impertinent* (Paris: JC Lattes), 1984.

5. Harry Beecher, *Experimentation in Man* (Springfield, MO: Charles C. Thomas), 1959. See also, Harry Beecher, "Ethics in Clinical Research," *New England Journal of Medicine*, June 16, 1966, vol. 274, no. 24, pp. 1354-1360.

6. Tom L. Beauchamp and James F. Children, *Principles of Biomedical Ethics* (New York: Oxford University Press), 1983. See also, Tom L. Beauchamp, *Case Studies in Business, Society, and Ethics* (Englewood Cliffs, NJ: Prentice Hall), 1983; and, Tom L. Beauchamp and Ruth Faden, eds., *Ethical Issues in Social Science Research* (Baltimore: Johns Hopkins University Press), 1982.

7. Conference Internationale des Ordres et des Organismes D'Attributions Similaires, "Principios de Etica Medica Europea," adopted Jan. 6, 1987.

8. Robert M. Veatch, "Against Virtue: A Deontological Critique of Virtue in Medical Ethics," in Earl E. Shelp, ed., *Virtue and Medicine* (Boston: D. Reidel Publishing Co.), 1985.

9. James McCartney, "Research on Children: National Commission Says 'Yes, If...,'" *Hastings Center Report*, vol. 8, Oct. 1978, pp. 26-31. Refers to the experiment conducted at Willowbrook State School, in which mentally retarded children were deliberately injected with the hepatitus virus. The purpose of the experiment was to see whether the disease could be better controlled in the institution. In response, the National Commission for the Protection of Human Subjects of Biomedical and Behavioral Research mandated guidelines to protect children from exploitation as research subjects. They reached a middle ground between a complete prohibition of research on children and an unqualified endorsement of research.

10. Leon Kass, *Toward a More Natural Science: Biology and Human Affairs* (New York: Free Press), 1985. The author talks about the need for such an approach; similar comments have been made by Richard McCormick, William F. May and Renee Fox.

Part I

The Character and Virtues of a Good Doctor

1.

Character, Virtue, and the Structure of the Doctor/Patient Relationship

Morality in the Medical Tradition

Professions have multiplied since the Middle Ages when the term, "profession," referred only to law, medicine, and priesthood. Now trades, businesses, and even salesmen form themselves into "professional" associations. The traditional groups, however, still constitute something of a paradigm for what the term profession means, and they demonstrate the critical importance of ethics for a true professional. Historically, what priests, doctors, or lawyers professed was an ethical reality: to hold themselves bound to do a certain type of good for others. They promised service and the many particular obligations which were listed in codes of professional conduct. The medical codes, for example, were simply a written expression of the moral obligations assumed by persons who "professed" to help those who were ill. A lived ethics, in the sense of a commitment to objective moral standards, constituted the essence of a profession.[1]

But professional claims of goodness today are suspect and open to criticism. Critics like Robert Veatch have pointed out the self-serving quality of some professional statements of service, as well as the "better than thou" attitude to which the professionals are often tempted. Inevitably, the professed ethics of a particular professional group will be a narrow and limited one. But do the limitations and justifiable criticisms negate the ethical substance of a profession like medicine? Max Weber, in his classical study of professions, did not think so. He recognized that economic considerations play an important role in medicine but do not exhaust the reality of doctoring. Those who look with cynicism at traditional medical ethics ignore the lived ethical reality which is still part of day-to-day medical practice. An objective morality of act analysis and rule creation leaves too much of what goes in medicine out of consideration.

Weighing the consequences of acts and creating norms of behavior in cases of conflict cannot be all there is to medical morality, and yet these concerns, as we have seen, have come to dominate the medical ethical landscape. As cultures move away from shared moral beliefs and common religious meanings, they move toward forms of unity based on procedural rules and norms alone. This has occurred in Western culture generally, and also in the medical profession. The loss of a fiduciary doctor/patient relationship associated with increased technology is taken to be a fact of contemporary life. Some doctors and many medical ethicists therefore feel comfortable with a more impersonal style of ethics, preferring to understand ethical responsibility in terms of legal contracts and agreed upon rules.

But most physicians can still relate to the traditional ethic. They want to be trusted by patients, to be loved by them and to conduct their lives so as to earn both. Even in our time, some of the older shared moral beliefs remain intact. Most modern doctors can identify with much of the spirit of traditional, professional codes and with the lived ethic or traditional virtues of older physicians. This older ethics, a more interior one, may be taken into account without denying more objective dimensions of the dominant style of today's medical ethics.

The ethical influence of physician models whom medical students emulate and imitate has not disappeared, and there is increasing attention being given to the character and virtue of applicants to medical specialties. In psychiatric residencies, for example, when there are more applicants than places available, a great deal of attention is given to the personal ethical qualities of applicants. An ethical review, in the sense of some assessment of moral character, will be carried out with more sophistication in some places than in others, but nowhere is it completely missing. Admissions committee members have an idea of the character and virtues needed to be a good doctor.

Even after medical training is finished, ethical training continues in a slightly different form. Certain medical virtues are cultivated by strong group sanctions against gross character deficiencies. If doctors do not attend to their patients or show some concern for the public image of the profession, they will be censured in subtle and sometimes unsubtle ways. Such doctors may survive in a time of scarcity or even prosper if they have exceptional technical talents, but a price is paid for violating an unspoken traditional ethics with its cornerstone in character and traditional virtues. If practicing physicians stray too far afield, they are likely to be in serious official trouble with the ethics board of the medical society or the review board of the hospital where they have privileges. Most assuredly, they will suffer from declining referrals from their fellow physicians.

Critics of the medical profession find it easy to ridicule this dimension of medical practice. For example, they see patients' trust in doctors, which medical training works to justify and engender, as a pure manipulation of patients for further economic gain. Correspondingly, patient trust according to some ethicists, undermines consumer self-protection, which is considered the essence of a good doctor/patient relationship. The effect of serious illness and fear of death are considered regrettable only because they diminish a patient's autonomy and power to contract. This style of criticism is too facile about assuming physician greed and reflects an ignorance of what it means to be ill. Just such an ignorance and an isolation from the clinical context stand behind some of the crusades for autonomy and contract models for medical ethics. On the other hand, the importance of virtue and character can also be exaggerated.

In the discussion of doctors' virtues which follows, there is no intent to reduce morality in the medical tradition to virtue and character formation. No suggestion is made that a medical ethics focusing on virtue should replace an ethics of rights, principles and duties. Ethics, as an enterprise striving to make sense out of the complexities of a lived moral life, needs many styles and emphases to do minimal justice to its objective. Virtue and rights, character and duty, principles and personality, all have a place in ethics, and, in fact, are all interrelated.

A Place for Ideals and Excellence

Virtue and character are neither purely subjective nor strictly ideal categories. Objective standards for both can be derived from the very nature of the doctor/patient relationship. Sometimes, however, these standards function as ideals, serving more as goals toward which human conduct points but never attains (except in instances of saintly and supererogatory acts). Although the distinction between concrete moral standards and ethical ideals is real, it is not always easy to draw the line between the two. Parents, for example, feel obligated to conduct which, outside the parental commitment, would certainly be an ideal form of love and care. The same is true of doctors who sometimes feel obliged to heroic conduct toward their patients and generally are obliged to higher virtue than a nonprofessional persons. Rather than being beyond human accomplishment, ideals are very much a part of even ordinary behavior, in that our ordinary acts are modified by that to which we aspire. Ideals impinge on life and this is especially true in medicine.

Every human being, for example, is under moral obligation to respect others, to help them, to keep promises and secrets, and to be truthful, but the doctor is obliged to go beyond normal expectations in relationships with patients. By profession, the doctor is bound to higher ideals and higher virtues because of the nature of the medical relationship. Not unlike what is expected of the priesthood, people rightly expect more of the doctor. Virtue is not disassociated from objective standards of conduct, but higher standards of professional conduct require higher virtue and greater personal effort in character formation.

Virtue considerations are justified today because many of the issues facing physicians do not lend themselves to objective analysis and discrete solutions. Many problems not only lack solutions, but draw doctors into moral situations in ways which cannot be sorted out with objective norms. Doctors have to take action in clinical situations without being able to identify all of the objective facts, let alone the objective rules for the right thing to do. Conflicts often develop within families and between families and doctors that simply cannot be solved by following set rules anymore than the problems of aging, or lost love, or death can be handled by rules or rights. These existential situations call for responses more along the line of cultivated attitudes, and habits; that is, virtue and character responses.

Virtue and character have a place in medical ethics also because of the size of today's health care institutions. Not only is responsibility often diffuse, but much bad behavior can easily elude rules and policy reviews. Rules and norms governing behavior in the clinical setting cannot begin to cover the many important contacts between doctor and patient.[2] Virtue has the added advantage of fostering good acts even when no one is watching or reviewing or regulating.

Not everything about a medical ethics which focuses on character and virtue is perfectly clear, but there is enough clarity to proceed in broad, general strokes toward outlining the content of such an ethics. When the theory of virtue and character is used as a lens through which to look at medicine, something worthwhile is brought into focus. Young doctors can profit by reading about the character styles and virtues of great doctors, and older doctors can renew earlier ethical ideals by doing the same. Because my intention is to provide the outline of a practical guide for doctors, I will not enter into a discussion of the conceptual problems which philosophers raise about character-based ethics. Nor will I do a character development for doctors, which is a medical educator's task. I believe that the project of laying the foundation of a traditional, medical ethics is important enough to be undertaken before everything about it satisfies the cultivators of conceptual clarity.

We know there are both good doctors and bad ones. We know too, that there are certain traits which almost everyone wants and expects to find in good doctors. And we know that some doctors are thoroughly committed to their professions—doctors to the root of their being, while others could just as well be stock brokers or automobile dealers. All of us know doctors who, in their manner and personal behavior, have met our needs as patients, and we have all known doctors who have failed us in that regard. People who feel cheated by certain doctors often learn that others have had similar experiences. Consistently good, as well as consistently bad behavior, we all know, is one of the realities of the world of medical practice. My intention is to look at this world a little more closely, in order to find reasons and explanations for what we all know to be true: that character and virtue considerations are important in medicine.

Virtue and character considerations, therefore, belong in medical ethics. Medicine as a profession is already a philosophical vision, and creates its own orientation to the world. Its essential acts (diagnosis, treatment, pain relief, function restoration, caring) have a recognizable structure, which serves as a standard for virtues. Certain habitual behaviors can be identified which contribute to the fulfillment of a doctor's professional commitment and meet the nearly universal expectations of people who are ill.

A Patient-Oriented Ethics

Even in ordinary language, we distinguish between the technically proficient physician and a good doctor. The latter designation we reserve for physicians who have developed a truly healing ethos or way of being. A good doctor certainly must satisfy the demands of technical competence, but in addition, he or she has to become the type of person to whom sick people can relate. The good doctor becomes good by developing those traits and habits which correspond to the specific needs of sick persons. The way illness is lived by patients and the needs it creates in them serves as the objective guide for a good doctor's character development. The standards of a doctor's goodness are dictated by the many dimensions of the doctor/patient relationship. Medical ethics, in this perspective, is tied to the experience of the person who is ill and the relationship between patient and healer.

The doctor/patient relationship has its own history, beginning with the Hippocratic physicians, passing through early medieval and modern Christianity, and ending in our own post-Christian secular era.[3] Each historical period brought changes, but most of what can be called the underlying structure of the doctor/patient relationship has remained the same.[4] Historical variations actually have made clearer certain basic characteristics about the way doctors relate to patients whom they try to help. Becoming aware of this enduring structure of the doctor/patient relationship is important because it sheds light on familiar routines and helps bring to them a higher moral tone. This structure is so full of personal elements that to ignore the personalistic dimensions of the doctor/patient relationship is to do violence to what ordinary medical practice is all about.

The plan of this study is to look at the various dimensions of the doctor/patient relationship and then to organize around its constitutive elements those personal moral characteristics which enable physicians to become good doctors in the sense of addressing all the needs of their patients. First, we will look at the project in outline form and then in subsequent chapters we will examine each element more carefully.

The Doctor/Patient Relationship

Outside the Medical School at the University of Madrid, a large sculpture depicts one human being bending over to help another who is obviously ill. This work of art was chosen because it was thought to capture what medicine is all about. The doctor/patient relationship is one in which the medical needs of one person and the technical ability of another form the basis of a humane partnership. Medicine is a form of human encounter characterized by help.

The doctor/patient relationship is more than a narrow professional concern because human beings are, by nature, indigent. Persons need help from others from the moment of birth to the time of death, but especially (and in a particular way) in times of illness. The doctor's help is called assistance, a term which in its etymological roots means "to stand alongside another (*ad-sistere*)." What the doctor does for the sick person involves, by definition, a certain closeness or relationship.

All who look at modern, high-tech medicine agree that this relationship is threatened. Technically-minded physicians have dreamed of a medical art devoid of relationship, and based entirely upon data provided by machines and computers. This view influences every aspect of high-tech medical care. Medical acts in this view not only could be carried out without doctor/patient contact, but in fact would best be carried out in a non-personal way. In a technical, medical utopia, sophisticated error-free tests linked with medical computer programs would eliminate the personal relationship between doctor and patient entirely, and it is claimed, improve the delivery of health care.

One hears less praise today for such utopian schemes than when they first emerged as possibilities. After years of experience, with sophisticated technology and doctors trained primarily in the non-human dimensions of medicine, medical educators have started trying to take some old humanistic elements in medical education out of storage. Postgraduate examinations in major medical specialties have begun to test for character traits in young doctors which enable them to enter real human relationships with patients. Because patients are biological and chemical, anatomical and physiological, an objective, impersonal, scientific medical approach is both understandable and necessary. But patients are also persons. Besides being organs, cells, bones, tissues and immune systems, they are intelligent, free, social, artistic and symbolic beings. Therefore, medical treatment has to be more than objective and scientific. Because patients have personalities, character, virtues, vices, fears, thoughts, projects and loves, these dimensions, too, have a place in the way they are treated by doctors.

In modern times, impersonal, technical developments abound, and consequently, the human dimension of medicine has come under considerable pressure. (Even psychiatric medicine, which in the psychoanalytic period became a refuge for the personal aspects of medical treatment, today has moved toward purely chemical, biological approaches.) New technologies separate doctors from their patients in even more subtle ways.[5] But just at the time when the personal elements of medicine are most threatened, they are also most missed, and demands are heard everywhere for their return.

Will medical authorities respond only by requiring testing for personal qualities in aspirants to medical schools? If so, nothing much will change. More structured approaches to virtue and character have to be given a place in medical education, and they must be solidly grounded approaches. The only realistic ground for a personalistic medical ethics is the structure of the doctor/patient relationship. An ethics of the inner person in the sense of a character and virtue-based medical ethics must start from the most basic concrete experience of medical practice. It has to be an existential ethics rooted in the lived experience of physicians and patients in relationship. This encounter, repeated over and over throughout the centuries, is the most permanent and the most universal medical reality and serves as the only ground on which a more personal medical ethics which aspires after objectivity can be built. The dimensions of this doctor/patient relationship are:

- Medical (diagnostic and therapeutic acts)

- Spiritual (the verbal communication between doctor and patient)

- Volitional (doctor and patient decisions)

- Affective (the feelings of doctors and patients for one another)

- Social (the broader, societal aspects of medical acts)

- Religious (doctors in some situations playing a priestly role)

Each dimension will be looked at in some detail. For now, it will suffice to show what these different dimensions of the doctor/patient relationship mean and how they will be used in this study.

I
The Medical Dimension

Every human relationship has its cognitive dimension and, in the medical encounter, this takes a specific form called diagnosis. It is the doctor who bears the major cognitive responsibility of knowing the patient in the sense of knowing what is wrong with him. The patient, of course, plays a role in this too because both have a stake in the doctor's coming to know what is wrong. Doctor and patient come together to know something that is important to both parties.

But what kind of knowledge is diagnosis? Is it a purely objective knowing of a passive object, not essentially different from the way physicists know the cosmos? Obviously not. Even in physics, there is the influence of the thing known on the knower and vice versa. But the "thing" in the case of medical diagnosis is no/thing. The person of the patient needs to be known because each patient's way of being has a crucial influence on whatever is wrong with him. Rather than being a purely objective scientific knowing, medical diagnosis is a personal meeting of two human beings. Good diagnosis involves a knowing of the patient as a person.

If medical diagnosis cannot occur outside a personal relationship between doctor and patient, neither can treatment. A famous German clinician used to tell his students that treatment begins when you shake hands with your patient. Good clinicians everywhere would endorse this idea as a shorthand formula for a larger truth: the person of the doctor, his presence, his character and his reputation all have an important effect on the patient's improvement. Another clinician put it this way: the doctor, himself, is the first medicine prescribed.

If diagnosis is fundamentally an interpersonal act, treatment is even more so. The doctor and patient must collaborate as persons in order to get the best therapeutic results. The doctor who treats the patient as an object and silently prescribes remedies for tissue or cell abnormalities not only violates the person of the patient, but reduces his therapeutic effectiveness. On the other hand, the doctor who takes the time to be involved with the person who is his patient is a better doctor in both a medical and an ethical sense.

The goal of therapy, of course, is restoration of health, a state not easy to define precisely because of its complexity. Because this is not a treatise on the philosophy of medicine, we will be satisfied here with an understanding which combines the objective and scientific with the subjective lived dimensions of medical well-being. Health, for our purposes, will be understood as a psychosomatic state of being in the service of a person's life and liberty. It will be taken to mean the physical capacities of the person to realize his life projects with a minimum of discomfort and, if possible, with satisfaction. Restoring health through the essential medical acts of diagnosis and treatment will require personal qualities which we will include under the virtue of *benevolence*.

II
The Spiritual Dimension

Speech has always been seen as something mysterious. *Nous* in Greek, and "symbol" in English both suggest a level of reality which is beyond the purely physical. Since speech is one of the uniquely human characteristics, it can be expected to play a role in the doctor/patient relationship. Good doctors speak to their patients just as any kind of good human help involves people talking to one another. The Good Samaritan surely did more than just provide physical help for the Jew in need along the road. Certainly they spoke to one another and exchanged personal information. The Samaritan would not have merited the qualifier, Good, if he had helped but never spoken or exchanged bits of personal information about himself, or inquired about the injured man's life.

What happens in any real helping has to happen in medicine. What comes to be known through diagnosis and the plans which are formulated for therapy must be shared with the patient in a way that is adequate to the patient's needs. The help which the patient seeks from the doctor is not exhausted in diagnosis and therapy. Illness creates a painful ignorance, and the patient wants the doctor to relieve that ignorance. Patients want to know what's wrong with them, what can be done to help, treatment options, alternatives, and more. Each patient has an individual set of questions which need to be discussed with the doctor. Even when diagnosis and therapy are successful, if doubts and questions are not addressed, patients go away unsatisfied. Doctors who do not talk to their patients fail in an important dimension of their medical responsibility. Medical assistance, therefore, involves verbal communication. We will discuss our attitudes or dispositions to communicate under the virtue of *truthfulness*.

III
The Volitional Dimension

Because they are persons, patients need help, and they need information, and they are condemned to make choices related to their illnesses. The responses which patients make to their illnesses and to the information they receive about them are never fixed or determined. A gap between the human person and his surroundings creates a pause out of which human persons formulate a response. Every truly human response is chosen and, therefore, carries with it reasons, motives, and purpose. Animals react to surroundings, but persons respond to an environment for their own reasons and their own ends.

What is true of human choices generally is true, as well, of the specific decisions to consent to or to refuse what the doctor suggests as treatment. If choosing is inevitably part of the doctor/patient relationship, it must be recognized and respected by both parties. Doctors choose to accept or not to accept a patient. Patients choose to respect the doctor's best judgment and the doctor must do the same for the patient. An essential dimension of a doctor/patient relationship is the disposition toward *respect* which each shows for the other's freedom.

IV
The Affective Dimension

The processes of diagnosis, therapy, verbal communication and choice all contribute toward the formation of a feeling bond between doctor and patient. It was Freud who noticed the special form of affection which patients develop for their doctors and vice versa. He called it "transference." Because psychoanalytic treatment involves discussion and a long term association, this affective dimension becomes more evident, but it is part of every doctor/patient relationship. This affection could be called love, but it would be a peculiar type of love. There are feelings associated with the doctor/patient relationship, but not the type of affect we ordinarily understand as love. In the doctor/patient relationship, each person contributes a different set of feelings. The patient brings his needs, expectations, confidence and admiration for the power of the doctor. The doctor contributes a desire to help the patient, a common human kindness and, possibly, an interest in money, fame or the domination of nature by his powers.

If love seems to be an inappropriate term for the feeling dimension of the doctor/patient relationship, friendship may be better in the sense of a unique medical friendship. Modern medical technicians may find such talk alien to their experience. It is not because affect and feelings are absent from their relationship, but because there is such emphasis on the technological and impersonal dimensions of healing that the personal feelings are not able to develop fully. Talk about the medical virtue of *friendliness* will attempt to re-emphasize this important aspect of doctoring.

V
The Social Dimension

Everything we have said about a doctor/patient relationship takes place within a certain social setting. Doctors and patients are not related as separate atoms, but as persons rooted in a complex of social realities. The human being, we know from the Greeks, is *zoon politikon* (a political being). Because human life requires a social context, the doctor/patient relationship has its own social dimension. It may seem as though the relationship is essentially private and its social context is limited to the small area of the doctor's office. But this is not true.

Illness is social in the sense that there are social causes of illness and social disabilities, and both may change from culture to culture. Illness makes a patient vulnerable in some social settings, and this is certainly true of the patient in a modern, high-tech hospital. Because the hospital is an alien environment, the patient does not know his way around, does not understand the procedures, and is unaware of who has power or how the power is used. Consequently, the doctor/patient relationship today creates a need on the part of the patient for help and protection against the worst social effects of illness, and assistance in gaining access to hospital help when it is necessary.

The doctor/patient relationship is social also in the sense that the patient comes from a certain socioeconomic condition, which may or may not provide equal access to the doctor's help (The very possibility of medical treatment is influenced by one's social situation). What the doctor does to the patient also has a social effect. In Greece during the fourth and fifth centuries B.C., whether a patient was a slave or a free man had a lot to do with the kind of medical treatment he received. In the final years of the twentieth century A.D., there is still a different medicine for the rich and the poor,[6] and this social dimension of the doctor/patient relationship calls for a personal response on the part of doctors, which will be discussed under the virtue of *justice*.

VI
The Religious Dimension

Human beings are structurally religious just as they are structurally needy, ethical, social, spiritual and affective. Even atheists are religious in the sense that all human beings form their lives on the basis of a vision of what life is all about, and the vision is always supported by faith instead of science. Some atheists may be very religious in that they are constantly preoccupied with that vision and its associated meanings. Less religious types make an effort to live day by day, attending only to what is at hand. But at certain times in life, the attachment to routine is broken, and ultimate questions force themselves into consciousness. Serious illness and imminent death are just such times, and consequently, doctors are often drawn into religious concerns.

Human beings also form images of themselves, and ordinarily the body is a ready instrument to pursue particular images. Individual goals and purposes reflect our self-images, and a healthy body permits their active pursuit. Bodily activity is an agent of personalized projects, and when illness occurs, life falls into turmoil. Serious illness threatens our images, purposes and goals, and so, threatens the very meaning of our lives. The body itself, which ordinarily is a ready instrument for other pursuits, becomes the focus of our attention. Patients rely on doctors in such a crisis, developing respect and affection for them, depending on them for information, looking to them for advice, orientation, protection, and perhaps even for help in deciphering the meaning of life and death.

Seriously ill and chronically ill patients suffer an assault upon their self-image and consequently, upon their identity and integrity. Often they look to the doctor for a way of coming to terms with the meaning of their lives in face of this change.[7] If death is imminent, questions about life's meaning may insert themselves into the doctor/patient relationship. The doctor's medical expertise does not make him an authority on religious issues, but neither can these issues be avoided in many doctor/patient encounters. When religious issues emerge within the doctor/patient relationship, the doctor may or may not address them. If the patient needs help with issues of ultimate meaning or struggles to hope when all human possibilities seem exhausted, at least the doctor has an opportunity to respond. Religion, as a virtue, is the personal quality which makes it possible for the doctor to be adequate to this last possible patient need.

Conclusion

Now that we have a general idea of the basic structure of the doctor/patient relationship, we can look at its constitutive elements in more detail. Our purpose is not to sound the depths of every aspect of this complex bond, but rather to identify those character traits of the physician which most adequately complement the different patient needs and best dispose the doctor to fulfill medical responsibilities which derive from them.

Elements which we have called diagnostic, therapeutic, symbolic, volitional, social, affective, and religious constitute the different dimensions of the bond between doctor and patient. To be a good doctor, modern physicians, like their historical Western predecessors, need personal qualities which enable them to be engaged fully with their patients. Technical mastery of non-human dimensions of illness is not enough. If only a part of the medical relationship is realized (the technical-scientific dimension), then something radically deficient occurs. If the medical act has human and technical dimensions, then the modern physician who is prepared to carry out only a part of the relationship is only partly prepared for medical practice. The adequate doctor needs a certain character formation which makes it possible to address the real needs of real patients.

Notes

1. Berlant, J.L., *Profession and Monopoly: A Study of Medicine in the United States and Great Britain* (Los Angeles: University of California Press), 1975.

2. Starr, P., *The Social Transformation of American Medicine: The Rise of a Sovereign Profession and the Making of a Vast Industry* (New York: Basic Books), 1982.

3. Lain Entralgo, Pedro, *La Relacion Medico-Enfermo* (Madrid: Alianza Editorial), 1983.

4. The Hippocratic Oath with some slight changes has endured for 2500 years, and spawned other codes which updated its norms from time to time. For a survey of this history, see "Code of Medical Ethics," *Encyclopedia of Bioethics,* Warren T. Reich, ed. (New York: The Free Press), 1978.

5. For a thorough analysis of the influence of technology on the practice of medicine, see Reiser, Stanley J., *Medicine and the Reign of Technology* (New York: Cambridge University Press), 1978; and Reiser, Stanley J., *The Machine at the Bedside* (New York: Cambridge University Press), 1984.

6. Iglehart, J., "Medical Care for the Poor: A Growing Problem," *New England Journal of Medicine,* 1985, 313:59.

7. Bernard, David, "The Physician as Priest Revisited," *Journal of Religion and Health,* vol. 24, no. 4, Winter, 1985.

2.

Diagnosis, Prognosis, and the Virtue of Benevolence

It is one thing to make a generic argument for the place of character and virtue in medical ethics and a more difficult thing to argue convincingly for those specific character traits which make a good doctor. It is one thing to insist on the place of a personal quality in the doctor/patient relationship and another thing to specify those particular personal qualities of a good practitioner. We have already rejected any listing of edifying traits as ineffective, and instead opted for developing a catalogue of character traits dictated by the needs of patients and the nature of medical acts. Since the quintessential medical acts are diagnosis and treatment, we look first to them to identify character traits which dispose doctors to meet the most basic patient needs and to satisfy to the fullest the calling of medicine.

That specific form of good (*bene*) which the doctor does (*facere*) for persons who are ill is summarized under the principle of *beneficence*. The principle of beneficence is to medicine what the principle of freedom is to journalism: the foundational ethical standard. The goods which are peculiar to medicine and which doctors publicly vow to accomplish, are precisely those referred to by this term: curing disease, relief of pain, restoring lost function, etc. Beneficence refers to goodness in the sense of diagnosis and treatment of illness. Above all else, the good doctor must carry out the basic medical acts. No other good equals this good. Beneficence, then, is the guiding principle of the medical professional, the constitutional ethical responsibility which first and above all else the doctor must strive to fulfill.

If beneficence is the objective ethical principle which refers to those good acts peculiar to medicine, benevolence is the virtue or character trait which disposes the doctor to carry out beneficent acts. Before the good (*bene*) can be done (*facere*), the good (*bene*) must be willed (*volere*). Bene/volence refers to the commitment or will to carry out medical acts according to the highest ethical standards. It refers to wishing (*volere*) a patient well or being disposed to attend to the patient's needs. Patients approach the doctor for a particular kind of help, and benevolence is the virtue which disposes the doctor to provide that help.

The medical help which patients need and doctors promise, must be effective, but effectiveness depends on more than technical medical competence. The virtue of benevolence disposes doctors to personal medical acts of diagnosis and prognosis. It refers to the doctor's continuing will to carry out diagnostic and therapeutic activities in more than a mechanically correct fashion. Rather than being just a nice addition to technical capacities, benevolence disposes the doctor to carry out the essential medical acts personally, as well as proficiently. It is the essential medical virtue.

Diagnosis and treatment are usually thought of as strictly technical operations. Doctors usually do not think about the many theoretical presuppositions which inform what superficially appear to be purely objective clinical determinations. "This is a case of cirrhosis," or, "you have kidney stones," or, "after discounting all other possibilities, I'd say that this is a case of genetically caused bipolar illness." Closer attention to "objective" clinical judgments, however, shows the influence of culturally approved theoretical paradigms on what appears to be purely objective findings. What one sees diagnostically in clinical medicine is, in large part, a function of assumed underlying theories. And medical paradigms of illness and disease have changed over the course of history. (Multiple sclerosis, for example, has been differently understood, and most recently is being conceptualized as an autoimmune disease). At the very least, the "purely objective" diagnostic acts are subjective in the sense of being influenced by moral evaluations.

Rarely is an individual patient nothing more than a typical case of a certain diagnostic category. The individual patient's life not only has something to do with the appearance of an illness, but personal attributes which patients bring to the diagnostic process also affect the form and content of the diagnosis. In other words, besides the subjective epistemological influences on medical acts, there are also influences coming from the personal dimension of the doctor/patient relationship. "Really?" a doctor might be compelled to ask. Can the quality of the patient's relationship with the doctor in any way affect a diagnosis of cancer or diabetes? In certain cases, obviously not, but in many diagnostic situations, the personal quality of the doctor/patient relationship can have a considerable influence on the outcome of a diagnosis.

For example, if the patient feels neither comfortable with nor accepted by a doctor, personal data that may be delicate and embarrassing but nevertheless very important for the diagnosis, will not be revealed. Lack of a good personal relationship will certainly affect the confidence which a patient develops in the doctor and this, in turn, can even affect the symptoms and the course of an illness. I personally know of many cases in which patients who finally got an appointment with Karl Menninger improved in anticipation of the visit with him; such was the effect upon their illness of an anticipated personal relationship with a trusted physician.

If a diagnosis is improved, and the symptoms of illness improve also as a result of a personal relationship with the doctor, how does the doctor develop the dispositions which foster this type of patient rapport? How does the doctor actually become benevolent? How does benevolence translate into a personalized form of medical help or into acts of personalized beneficence? How does benevolence dispose the doctor to make a diagnosis of the person as a patient, rather than a reductionistic one involving only tissues and organs? How does it dispose the doctor to a relationship with the whole patient rather than just a partial or even dehumanizing contact? And how do such personalized medical acts differ from impersonal or a-personal ones?

The virtue of benevolence translates into those characteristically human acts associated with the beginnings of a genuine medical relationship. Patients are neither biological specimens in which anatomic or physiological abnormalities occur, nor biological battlegrounds where microbes struggle with leukocytes and antibodies. Patients live their illnesses, feel them, develop attitudes toward them, like rebellion, resignation, terror. They try to find messages in them like punishment, opportunity, test. They are either afraid or not, confident of getting better, or in a state of despair. The benevolent doctor does not merely strive to make an objectively valid diagnosis, but rather a personalized objective one. Since the illness is a lived reality, its lived dimension figures in the fuller picture. Benevolence disposes the doctor to this lived reality, and thereby, to both a more human and more objectively correct diagnosis.

The benevolent doctor acts differently from a colleague who thinks of himself and of medicine in purely impersonal terms. Benevolence creates openness to the patient's lived experiences and interest in what the patient has to say about his illness. It does not mean that the doctor shares the patient's aches and pains, but it does mean that he takes an interest in the way the patient reacts to this pain or lives a particular diagnosis. If the benevolent doctor cannot find objective indications of illness (for example, a sciatic pain), he does not assume immediately that there is no illness or that the patient is simulating. (It may be that there is simulation, but that judgment does not follow immediately from the failure to find objective clinical signs.) Benevolence disposes the doctor to take the patient's personal experience seriously and to try to work with the patient's experiences, even in the absence of objective verifications. Benevolent doctors, for example, do not make the mistake of confusing neurotic symptoms with simulations. In one, there is real suffering; not so in the other. In short, benevolence disposes the doctor to take an interest in the way physical abnormalities are reflected in personal experience, and humanizes the medical act of discovering the source of a patient's complaints.

We can summarize the various elements of the medical diagnosis in a simple diagram.[1]

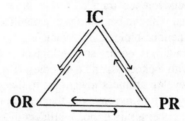

IC refers to the immediate cause of illness: external cause (trauma, microbe, poison) and internal disposing cause (organic constitution, psychic or somatic condition).

OR refers to the organic reaction to the immediate cause: the psychic, as well as somatic reaction which is determined by the patient's constitution. A patient's specific condition is determined by age, sex, race, biotype, biological past, immunological competency, hypersensitivity, etc.

PR refers to the personal reaction of a particular human being to all of the above. This personal response is influenced by the lived experiences of patients, their character, personal beliefs, sense of personal self, social situation, personal projects, individual biography.

The arrows pointing toward each point of the triangle indicate the relations among these three dimensions of an illness. The immediate cause (IC), influences both the organic reaction (OR) and the personal response (PR). The organic reaction and the personal response certainly act upon each other, and both, in turn, have an effect upon the immediate cause.

Medical diagnosis is nothing more or less than the most adequate or precise understanding of the dynamics of an illness, so as to be able to identify the proper nosological category, along with the individualized dimension of this particular incidence. There is an individual and personal dimension to a diagnosis (sometimes more important than others), and for this reason, benevolence, which disposes the doctor toward the person of the patient and personalizes the diagnostic task, belongs to the very substance and structure of what a good doctor does.

The good diagnostician is one who is adequate to every dimension of an illness: both a technically competent and a benevolent doctor. Benevolence, we repeat, disposes the self of the doctor to the needs of the patient who is a person and not just a body. It opens the doctor to the lived experience, personal intimacies, personal concerns, personal needs, personal fears, and to a recognition that they are all connected with the patient's illness.

Obviously, benevolence is the character trait that patients most want and expect in a doctor—a personal caring and an openness to real relationship. It creates the condition for the possibility of a doctor/patient relationship which is what it ought to be: a humane relationship rather than a dehumanizing, reductionistic one, no matter how scientifically sophisticated. This virtue both precedes a good diagnosis and creates the necessary condition for the possibility of practicing good medicine.

Benevolence in Therapy

If diagnosis is reduced to a purely technical analysis of the patient's somatic disturbance, treatment may correspondingly be reduced to a purely technical manipulation of the same partial dimension of the person who is ill. The medical treatment associated with an abstract or reductionistic view of the patient becomes a type of engineering. The early Freud thought of himself as an "engineer of the libido," and provides us with a good example of this reductionistic and impersonal attitude toward treatment. Later on, in his mature years, Freud developed a more adequate view of illness and a more personalized form of treatment. Modern medical training and practice seem to condition doctors in the direction of the early Freud and make the development of genuine personal relationships with patients very difficult. The all important technical understanding of an illness displaces that other understanding, which is equally important, and keeps the doctor from becoming a technician.

Diagnosis and treatment are medical acts which take place within a relationship between two complete persons rather than between a body and a scientific intelligence. Diagnosis and treatment are cognitive and operative dimensions of the doctor/patient relationship, which is inter/personal in its generic form and then becomes a specialized form of personal helping. Like diagnosis, treatment also involves personal elements. Because treatment, like diagnosis, occurs within a fully human relationship, to ignore the personal dimension of treatment is to impoverish this critical medical act.

Treatment is the principle help which doctors offer, not to a disease but to a patient; not a patient in general or to someone with this insurance policy or to number 29 on today's list, but to patient Bill Miles or Patty McMoran who sought out Dr. Woollcott's help for their particular problems. Bill and Pat bring themselves as persons with their individual biographies, needs, concerns, hopes, projects, and their individual forms of trust. Dr. Woollcott in turn, after taking into account and responding to the personal dimensions of their illness, directs his treatment to them as persons.

Of course, this ideal is not always realized. The patient can be treated purely and simply as a thing, on which proven remedies are applied. When this happens, the patient is turned into a reacting organism and the doctor into a technical manager of therapeutic properties. A more modern fall from the ideal would turn the doctor into a computer program operator who punches in test results and reads out prescriptions. To be fair, it must be admitted that these reductionistic views of doctor and patient relationships stand behind important advances of modern medicine. Precisely because of impressive results, these views have become dogma in some sectors of the medical community. For these "dogmatic doctors," any "weakening" of the hard nosed, scientific perspective with ethical and humanistic influences is anathema. Moral and humanistic considerations are taken to be enemies of science.

Scientific dogmas can be maintained only by wearing thick blinders and even ignoring much of what comes into view. The personal influence of the doctor is so powerful that it sometimes has a greater therapeutic effect on patients than sophisticated medicines. The placebo effect is one extrascientific reality which cannot be ignored, even by rigid scientific practitioners. I already mentioned the patient who improved after being accepted for an appointment with Karl Menninger or felt considerably improved after a single visit with him. Finally, who can ignore the tremendous importance of the patient's subjective attitudes on the outcome of treatment; the difference between the patient who really wants to get better versus the patient who knowingly or unknowingly has taken refuge in his symptoms?

Even the dogmatic doctor—the believer in a narrow scientific view of medicine—is constantly making medical decisions which can never be defended as scientific. In the absence of hard diagnostic data of proven results with a certain treatment, he or she would logically have to stop treating. Confronted with refractory illnesses, a hard-nosed scientific attitude would move toward a therapeutic nihilism. Ordinarily, however, doctors treat, follow hunches, rely upon anecdotal accounts of other physicians, and try to make up for the lack of scientific evidence with reasonable, but not proven, procedures.

Even less attractive than the positivistic practitioner is the avaricious doctor whose dominant concern is not scientific rigor, but monetary gain. Here, the lack of concern for the personal dimension of treatment leads to "therapeutic furor"; the opposite of therapeutic nihilism. The positivistic doctor may use non-scientific approaches without letting himself recognize the implication of his actions. The avaricious doctor, however, knows what he is doing, and has to repress the moral implications of his actions.

In the history of medicine, medical treatment has had its more personal periods and its less personal ones, and even today, with all the impersonal pressures, treatment in most cases turns out satisfactorily. But more attention to the personal could be more effective, as well as more humanizing for doctor and patient alike. Many bad feelings which patients harbor even after successful treatment could be avoided. Simulated benevolence which sometimes substitutes for personal treatment usually does not reach the corruption of total simulation and even manages to bring about a low level of personal treatment. The truth is that passage from a technically correct but impersonal treatment to a truly benevolent one is not difficult. Human beings, uncorrupted by narrow dogmas and with normal emotional development, naturally relate to others as persons. Doctors are not exceptions to this rule.

This is especially true in chronic rather than acute illnesses. The distinction is an old one in medicine and was supported by Sydenham and others on purely biological grounds. For our purposes, biography will do. We will call *acute* those illnesses which are felt to be temporary interruptions in the normal life of the patient and have not been incorporated definitively into the patient's way of being. The day after the flu, a person returns to his work and normal way of life. *Chronic* illness is the opposite. For the person with chronic asthma or chronic anything, the illness becomes integrated into the patient's lifestyle: it becomes his illness and part of his or her self-experience.

It is much easier for the doctor treating an acute illness to get away with a technically competent but non-benevolent posture. Without even looking into the patient's face or exchanging a verbal pleasantry, a doctor can recognize certain bacterial infections and simply apply an effective antibiotic. In some instances, a patient will be better in a matter of hours and nothing benevolent or personal will have taken place. As medical treatments become more and more effective, it becomes easier for doctors to adopt impersonal styles and to act more like biological engineers. All the more reason then, to ask if this should really be the way medicine is practiced. If the doctor, by being benevolent, can treat the whole person, increase the effectiveness of the medications, prevent psychic scars, and avoid malpractice claims, then why shouldn't benevolence be the virtuous disposition demanded by objective ethical standards of medical practice?

Besides, at some point, the most efficacious treatments in the world will fail. At some point, the doctor will not be able to cure. Does he or she then abandon the scene and turn the patient over to more humane professionals who know how to care, relieve and console? Not many years ago, the doctor would be expected to be at the bedside of dying persons. This is less and less the case today. Cancer patients who have been intensely involved with their doctors for long periods not only die without them, but live their final days and weeks without their company. At some point, the doctors or the family decide that "nothing more can be done" and, from that time on, many doctors disappear. What a shame! Is there really "nothing more that can be done"? The benevolent doctor can do much for the dying patient. An ethical self, formed by benevolence, can continue to help a patient even when powerful medications become useless. A benevolent doctor is disposed to remain with the dying patient, and is willing and able to offer therapeutic words when therapeutic procedures have become useless.

With chronically ill patients, it is difficult to be an effective doctor without benevolence. The illness's duration and the corresponding prolongation of the doctor/patient relationship means that either a personal dimension develops or treatment degenerates. As in a marriage without caring, in a purely technical, medical relationship both partners become miserable. Chronic illness will not even be adequately understood, let alone adequately treated without attention to more than biological factors. Either there will be a psychological factor in the emergence of the illness, or one will certainly develop when symptoms become personally appropriated. Illness and even pain can come to be somewhat satisfying or used for sympathy, or as an excuse not to work. Doctors who do not enter a personal relationship with chronically ill patients cannot treat them competently. The virtue of benevolence is required of the good doctor in either an ethical or technical sense of good.

If curing the chronic illness is not a real possibility, then the doctor will have to help patients do the best they can within the limits imposed by the illness. The patient's life will have to be reordered; perhaps a different style of life will have to be created. Treatment of this sort leaves no alternative to a doctor/patient relationship characterized by benevolence. Patients will have to share intimate details of changes effected by the chronic illness, and the doctor will have to enter into an appreciation of these personal dimensions in order to understand what will improve the patient's life. Doctors and patients, in effect, will have to cooperate in constructing a different lifestyle, and this requires an involvement in the most personal dimensions of the patient's life. Helping the chronically ill patient requires a doctor who is ethical in the sense of having developed a certain inner way of being rather than of knowing how to solve dilemmas. The doctor treating a chronic illness is forced to recognize that illness has personalized dimensions and that good doctors open their very being not just to an illness, but to a person who needs help. All this takes a certain type character.

Treating a chronic patient can be compared to the cooperation needed for sailing. In a small two-person sailboat, each crew member must know the other, care about him, and cooperate in refined and intimate ways to make the boat go. The illness is like a storm which brings adverse conditions. To make even the most modest progress against head-winds, the crew has to tack. The doctor is the captain who decides to try a certain maneuver. He and the patient have to be in close communication to get the most out of the equipment without forcing it beyond its limits. They go in one direction for awhile and then "turn about" to another. The shared, therapeutic goal functions as a rudder, and the doctor tries first one tack and then another, with the patient always feeding back information and participating in every decision to change course. No decision brings great progress, but the doctor remains firm and determined to make whatever progress possible against the wind. The doctor tries to keep alive a hope that some major environmental change will make the difficult cooperative project a little easier. The patient's feedback about how he feels provides the data on which treatment decisions (whether to continue in one direction or to change course) are made. Treatment is always difficult in chronic illness, and no progress is possible without the closest personal cooperation between doctor and patient. The good doctor needs to be ethical in the sense of being the type of person who can establish and retain such a rapport.

Summary

We have already made reference to the many obstacles thrown up by contemporary culture to considerations of character and the development of virtue. The personal relationship that should characterize the contact between patient and doctor is often difficult to establish. Some manage a refined development of benevolence and some do not. Even when the doctor makes an effort to be benevolent, the desired personal relationship, for one reason or another, may simply not develop. Human beings rarely reach the ideal and sometimes do not even manage the minimum conditions for being personal.

Certain classic obstacles are frequently implicated in the misfiring of the development of benevolence or a misfiring of its actualization in a particular case. A thoroughly scientific set of beliefs about the practice of medicine influences a doctor's character by creating a disposition toward the purely objective dimensions of illness. Such a doctor may be a good diagnostician and therapist in the all important technical aspects of these acts, but not a good doctor in a complete sense. Rather than benevolence, the dominant character traits of such doctors are scientific rigor and discipline.

Other doctors are consumed by even less noble interests and moral dispositions. The doctor dominated by greed, for example, can be a good technician and may even develop certain superficial personal forms of contact with patients as a way of generating income. But if the dominant character trait is covetousness, then every patient will be seen as an opportunity for gain, rather than as someone in need. This attitude disposes to maltreatment in the sense of overtreatment and other types of patient manipulation. Even more than a dominant scientific spirit, the spirit of covetousness undermines the essential medical virtue of benevolence.

More and more physicians today, not just in our culture, but all over the world, have become functionaries either of the state or of some other enterprise. The functionary also tends to develop certain character traits: he cares only about performing his function or doing his job and doing just enough to meet the minimum demands of the employer. The interest of the bureaucratic doctor shifts from the patient to the job requirements. Anyone who has ever lived in a socialist country or who has had to deal with capitalist bureaucracies, knows how people are treated by bureaucrats and how that treatment is neither benevolent nor personal. When bureaucratic treatment occurs in medicine, it leaves the recipient angry and dissatisfied.

All of the above mentioned attitudes toward medical practice are easily recognized as alternatives to the ideal we are describing with the principle of beneficence and the corresponding virtue of benevolence. Being benevolent is not only difficult in itself, but increasingly more difficult in an impersonal culture. For this reason, today's doctors who are convinced that the classical moral ideals of good medicine are valid have to work harder in order to be good. At the very least, being aware of the obstacles and temptations makes the development of a totally unbenevolent character less likely. That, in itself, is already a moral accomplishment.

Notes

1. Lain Entralgo, Pedro. *La Relacion Medico-Enfermo,* (Madrid: Alianza Editorial), 1983, p. 398. Other works include Lain Entralgo, Pedro. *Antropologia de la Esperanza.* (Madrid: Guadarrama), 1978; Lain Entralgo, Pedro. *Antropologia Medica Para Clinicos.* (Barcelona: Salvat), 1984; Lain Entralgo, Pedro. *Descargo de Conciencia.* (Barcelona: Barral Editores), 1976; Lain Entralgo, Pedro. *El Diagnostico Medico: Historia y Teoria.* (Barcelona: Salvat Editores), 1982; Lain Entralgo, Pedro. *Doctor and Patient.* (New York: McGraw-Hill), 1969; Lain Entralgo, Pedro. *El Medico en la Historia.* (Madrid: Taurus Ediciones), 1958; Lain Entralgo, Pedro. *Enfermedad y Pecado.* (Barcelona: Ediciones Toray), 1961; Lain Entralgo, Pedro. *Estudios de Historia de la Medicina y de Antropologia Medica.* (Madrid: Ediciones Escorial), 1943; Lain Entralgo, Pedro. *Grandes Medicos.* (Barcelona: Salvat), 1961; Marias, Julian. *Historia de la Filosofia y de la Ciencia: Julian Marias y Pedro Lain Entralgo.* (Madrid: Guadarrama), 1964; Lain Entralgo, Pedro. *Historia de la Medicina Moderna y Contemporanea.* (Barcelona: Editorial Cientifico Medica), 1963; Lain Entralgo, Pedro. *Introduccion Historica al Estudio de la Patologia.* (Madrid: Paz Montalvo), 1950; Lain Entralgo, Pedro. *Joaquin Albarran en la Historia de la Medicina.* (Madrid: S.N.), 1961; Lain Entralgo, Pedro. *La Amistad Entre el Medico y el Enfermo en la Edad Media: Discurso leido el dia 7 de junio de 1964, en su Recepcion Publica.* (Madrid: Alonso), 1964; Lain Entralgo, Pedro. *La Espera y la Esperanza: Historia y Teoria del Esperar Humano.* (Madrid: Revista de Occidente), 1957; Lain Entralgo, Pedro. *La Historia Clinica: Historia y Teoria del Relato Patografico.* (Madrid:Consejo Superior de Investigaciones Cientificas), 1950; Lain Entralgo, Pedro. *La Medicina Hipocratica: Estudio Preliminar de Pedro Lain Entralgo.* (Madrid: C.S. de I.C.), 1976; Lain Entralgo, Pedro. *La Universidad, el Intelectual, Europa: Meditaciones Sobre le Marcha.* (Madrid: Ediciones Cultura Hispanica), 1950; Lain Entralgo, Pedro. *Maranon y el Enfermo.* (Madrid: Revista de Occidente), 1962; Lain Entralgo, Pedro. *Menendez Pelayo y el Mundo Classico: Pedro Lain Entralgo.* (Madrid: Taurus), 1963; Lain Entralgo, Pedro. *Mind and Body, Psychsomatic Pathology: A Short History of the Evolution of Medical Thought.* (London: Harvill), 1955. Lain Entralgo, Pedro. *Mis Paginas Preferidas.* (Madrid: Editorial Gredos), 1958; Lain Entralgo, Pedro. *Mysterium Doloris: Hacia una Teologia Cristiana de la Enfermedad.* (Madrid: Publicaciones de la Universidad Internacional Menendez Pelayo), 1955; Lain Entralgo, Pedro. *Obras.* (Madrid: Editorial Plenitud), 1965; Lain Entralgo, Pedro. *Panorama Historico de la Ciencia Moderna.* (Madrid: Ediciones Guadarrama), 1963; Lain Entralgo, Pedro. *Sante et Maladie.* (Paris: Robert Laffont-Grammont), 1976; Lain Entralgo, Pedro. *Sobre la Universidad Hispanica.* (Madrid: Ediciones Cultura Hispanica), 1953; *Sydenham: Estudio Preliminar de Pedro Lain Entralgo y Agustin Albarracin Teulon.* (Madrid: C.S. de I.C.), 1961; Lain Entralgo, Pedro. *Teoria y Realidad del Otro.* (Madrid: Revista de Occidente). 1961; Lain Entralgo, Pedro. *The Therapy of the Word in Classical Antiquity.* (New Haven: Yale University Press), 1970; Lain Entralgo, Pedro. *Vida y Obra de Guillermo Harvey.* (Madrid: Espasa-Calpe), 1948.

3.

Medical Communication and the Virtue of Truthfulness

Benevolence, which disposes the doctor to the uniquely beneficent acts of medicine, obviously is not the only virtue of the good physician. Other virtues are required by other dimensions of the doctor/patient relationship. One might understand all other virtues as aspects of a truly benevolent attitude or rather as separate virtues corresponding to different dimensions of the medical relationship. Whether these other dimensions are separate but related or actually one reality with different forms is a theoretical question which lies outside the scope of this essay. For pragmatic reasons, I'll consider the different dimensions of the doctor/patient relationship to constitute separate foundations for different but related virtues. As the reader will recall, the underlying philosophical assumption of this essay is that the very structure of the doctor/patient relationship provides the objective ground for those moral attitudes and character traits which make for a good doctor. "Good," in this phrase, means several things: a doctor who treats patients the way they should be treated; one who addresses the needs which patients bring to the doctor; one who fulfills a publicly proclaimed medical vow to help persons who are ill; one who does what the doctor/patient relationship requires.

Being a good doctor in the above sense is harder than ever before. Doctors cannot help being upset about the cost of their malpractice insurance and all the paperwork required to practice medicine. Avaricious lawyers and ridiculous jury decisions certainly play a part, but do not completely explain the problem. It is neither an exaggeration nor an oversimplification to say that the malpractice crisis is the economic reflection of a deeper crisis in the doctor/patient relationship. An absence of attention to doctor virtues and character development has had a negative effect on many aspects of the doctor/patient relationship, but especially on the communication process. Many a lawsuit begins with a patient who is angry and dissatisfied about his or her doctor's lack of affability. The word affable in English comes from the Latin *ad fari* meaning "to speak to."

Technology has also contributed to the problem. How can doctors work with technology, be surrounded by machines, rely more and more on the data which they generate, and yet avoid loss of affability? This one influence, joined with overcrowded schedules, high patient loads, and unconcern about medical virtues, has led to increases in curt, incomprehensible, hurried, and downright unaffable communications with patients. Bad habits of communication both result from and play a role in bad character development, and the doctor, without even knowing it, comes to be an unaffable person. If bad communication occurs with your garbage collector or paper carrier, that's one thing. But when it is with your doctor, frustration of the worst kind occurs. And as a matter of statistical fact, well over 75 percent of all patients sampled in one survey reported just this high degree of frustration with their physicians.[1,2] They reported being interrupted consistently, not being allowed to finish accounts of their complaints, not having their questions answered, and in general, not being talked to properly.

If, over the years doctors have become bad communicators, over the years they can become more affable. This one ethical change could have a more salutary effect on the malpractice crisis than far more expensive insurance policies. If we consider talking to be spiritual in the sense that meaning borne by the sounds and symbols of language goes beyond purely physical, measurable, scientific reality, then we could say that a major threat to contemporary medicine's good health could be cured with a dose of spirituality.

Importance of Communication

More than once, we have talked of the doctor/patient relationship as a human contact first and then a particular type of personal meeting. As in every human relationship, there is in the doctor/patient relationship a communicative dimension. Diagnosis and treatment may be conducted via technological tests and in silence, but these acts reach their natural conclusion in a verbal communication between doctor and patient. Diagnosis and treatment plans need to be shared before they can be said to be complete. It is not enough for the doctor to know what is wrong with the patient and to plan to address the problem. The patient, too, needs to know about his or her condition. Being ill raises all sorts of questions that only a doctor can answer, and to leave the patient suspended before these pressing existential concerns is not only to leave the essential medical process incomplete, but to cause unnecessary pain.

Questions raised by illness inevitably suggest answers in the form of lay interpretations. Patients not only question, but make some types of diagnostic interpretations themselves. "This started because I was under pressure." "It was a certain meal I ate which caused the problem." "I think it must be cancer because my mother had cancer." "It seems to me that it is my heart." The communication of the doctor's diagnosis is often a reinterpretation of a lay diagnosis which calls for correction and alteration. Doctors who do not talk to patients or do not talk enough, leave the patient with all sorts of mistaken notions; the diagnostic process is left incomplete and therapeutic effectiveness is curtailed.

As free and self-actualizing beings, patients must participate in their treatment. To treat human beings without their participation or without communication with them is to treat them as objects. What Plato said about the silent treatment of slaves as opposed to medical treatment of free men in Ancient Greece is as true today as it was 2500 years ago. The treatment of free human beings requires communication and participation, and to do otherwise is to reduce the patient to the status of slave. Not to communicate is to deprive the patient of information required to participate freely and rationally in treatment decisions. The very structure of the doctor/patient relationship requires that disclosure and participation be carried out with sensitivity to the needs and interests of patients. A treatment plan must be directed to this particular patient, suffering this illness, in this particular way, interrupting this or that vital project, complicating a family or social situation, raising special psychological or religious problems. The corresponding disclosure then, has to be personal. The illness is like a storm which brings adverse conditions. And talking or not talking to patients in a personal way about questions they have regarding their illness is a matter of habit. Some doctors develop virtues of communication and some develop vices. Doctors who habitually give patients the silent treatment lack an essential medical character trait. They fall below the standards for good physicians.

A purely scientific doctor, interested primarily in an objective understanding of a somatic abnormality, will be tempted either to disclose nothing, or to disclose too little, or to disclose the truth in scientific jargon without making an effort to translate this information into something understandable to the patient. The assumption is that illness is nothing more than a bio-chemical abnormality which is fixed like any other mechanical problem. Either the doctor knows how to fix the illness or he doesn't. Talk and communication do not really count.

The avaricious doctor may tend to talk to patients if, by doing so, he thinks he can impress them or advance his reputation and correspondingly his income. But what he says may be intended primarily to please or impress rather than to communicate the truth. His talk tends to be insincere and, therefore, neither completes the diagnosis nor contributes to the patient's rightful participation in treatment decisions.

The physician functionary, whose patients are tasks which have to be taken care of, is inclined to say little, or to say what is required in a way that ignores the personal situation of the patient. The bureaucrat or functionary not only tends to see little in his diagnosis, but to say little about what he has found. "I think you will be all right." or "I don't find anything." The functionary's concern is to get finished with work and to get home. Talking to patients just extends the workday, something to be avoided at all costs.

Obviously, the ideal forms of doctor/patient communication are related to benevolence. The benevolent physician who truly opens himself to the needs of his patient will be most disposed to take the time to communicate and to be truthful in his communication. Benevolence disposes doctors to personal execution of the medical acts, and such execution includes a dimension of personalized truthful communication. Truthfulness is a virtue corresponding to the communicative dimension of the doctor/patient relationship, and truthfulness is obviously related to benevolence.

What the Patient Communicates

In valid communication between doctor and patient, each party talks and each tells the truth. Patients talk about themselves, their illness, events related to their illness, and their interpretation of the illness. Patients also talk about whatever else in their lives they see as related to the illness. Patients describe their experiences as patients (from *patior, pati, passus,*—to suffer) in contrast to their experience as agents (from *ago, agere actus*—to act). They observe and interpret the symptoms of illnesses which they are undergoing or suffering. Patients are both witnesses and exegetes of their infirmity. All of this they relate to the doctor. What one notices in the talk of patients is a personalized and utterly truthful account of illness: the way illnesses are lived and affect their lives.

Patients talk about their world: their work, their projects, their circumstance, in the sense that the Spanish philosopher Ortega y Gassett uses that term when he says "I am myself and my circumstance" (*Yo soy yo y mis circumstancias*). Patients talk about their bodies: red spots on the skin, swollen ankles, headaches, pains in the chest, weakness, diarrhea, etc. They talk about the sadness, fears, hopes and despairs associated with their illness. And, finally, they talk about their own interpretations of all of this.

A doctor's interruptions, interjections and questions originate in an attempt to translate this personalized data into a more objectified scientific language. "Would you describe the pain as sharp?" "Did it move down your arm?" "Did you feel anything in your jaw?" "Did it subside when you sat down?" "Did it feel as though someone were grabbing you in the middle of the chest or as though someone were sitting on your chest?" Once the lived experience of the symptoms is given a form that makes it fit into the doctor's way of understanding things, the doctor can move either to a correction or a confirmation of the almost inevitable patient interpretation of the illness.

What patients say obviously has an importance for the process. The act of talking to the doctor about an illness has other functions as well. Talking with the doctor, the patient moves into the personal space opened up for him by the benevolent physician. The listening doctor, in a sense, accompanies the patient as the story of his passage from health to illness is told. The patient's story is like a confession, and in getting it off of his chest, the patient feels relief. There is also a clarification and a psychological ordering of the material which occurs as the patient tells his story to the doctor. Sometimes, the patient's account contributes to a sense of personal importance as the doctor listens with rapt attention, listening as few persons have ever listened.

Both what the patient says and the fact that he says it are important. When the benevolent physician opens himself to the patient and the patient responds to this invitation with the true story of his illness, a new note is added to the doctor/patient relationship and a new depth is achieved.

What Doctors Say

Doctors do not talk about themselves. They, too, talk about the patient and the patient's illness. The doctor asks questions, sometimes very personal ones, about the symptoms and the patient's life, which help him to move the patient's talk into his own categories. For this reason, doctors frequently ask patients to tell them more about some detail or another of the story, and doctors provide encouragement and clarification and explanations of what they believe is going on in the patient. If substantial doubt about the diagnosis remains, truthfulness requires that this too be talked about, as well as all the medically acceptable options which are available to the patient, including the option of no treatment when this is realistic.

The content of the doctor's talk, as well as its style and sensitivity, is influenced by the virtue of benevolence in the sense that talk about diagnosis and treatment (like these medical acts themselves) gives expression to a genuine, human relationship with the patient. What the doctor says is a verbal manifestation of benevolence: the doctor's willingness to help the patient in both physical and spiritual ways.

Truthfulness, however, is the virtue which disposes the doctor to carry on the kind of communication appropriate to this dimension of the doctor/patient relationship. What the doctor says is a truthful response to the interest, questions, needs and concerns of the patient. We will talk more about what truthfulness requires below, but here it might be appropriate to mention that truth, as we are using it, is more closely tied to beauty than to crude factual communication. When some people preface a remark with a phrase like "I am going to tell you the truth," they are usually about to say something hurtful. Truth is often linked with aggression. The truth which the physician communicates, however, is closer to what Plato talked about as *logos kalos,* beautiful talk.[3] The virtue of truthfulness in the physician disposes to a real communication designed to meet the patient's needs, and to a beautiful communication in the sense of being a sensitively and artfully delivered truth. This type of truthfulness can be learned. And the art can become part of a doctor's character. After all, the doctor, like every other human being, is naturally affable.

One final point. When the doctor speaks truthfully to the patient, the communication acquires a sacral character. What the doctor says, like the divine word or the words of Adam naming things in the Genesis story, creates a reality for the patient and, at the same time, exercises power over that reality. What the doctor says has power to change the patient, sometimes in very substantial ways—all the more reason why more attention should be given to communication and dispositions to communicate. This virtue, however, is not always in the form of speech.

Silence and Talk

Human beings are, at one and the same time, the only animals who talk and the only ones who keep silent (*Animal loquax et simul taciturnum*). Silence makes no sense in reference to non-talking animals. In silence as well as in talk, humans communicate symbolically; that is, with added meaning. Silence provides both the ground out of which speech arises and an opportunity for someone to speak. It also constitutes the only appropriate response to certain situations. Ludwig Wittgenstein, the Oxford philosopher, expressed this idea in his usual, succinct way: "Where one cannot speak, thereof one must be silent."[4]

In the face of death and tragedy, God and mystery, humans adopt silence because the reality is beyond words. Words always have a certain inadequacy about them, and as the realities faced become more serious, words become less and less adequate. At some point, words become inappropriate, and silence becomes the only adequate form of expression. Doctors appropriately adopt silence in the face of terrible loss or in the face of death. At such points, a benevolent silence is the only appropriate communication. The virtue of truth, in the face of mystery, takes the form of silence. Doctors often find themselves in such situations, and therefore, the good doctor, besides knowing how to talk truthfully, also knows how to be silent. Patients do not have to learn silence, and many use this form of communication. There are times for both the patient and the doctor when silence both carries deep meaning and is an appropriate expression of truth.

But not all silence falls into this category. Sometimes, patients are silent simply because they do not understand what is going on. Rather than being an appropriate response to an ineffable reality, sometimes silence simply means "I don't understand" or "I don't know what to say." When doctors confront this type of silence, they need to try again to communicate with the patient. Another silence is of the "I don't want to talk" type—a silence of aggression rather than of ignorance. Many psychiatric patients adopt silence as their armament against a doctor whom they hate. Silent aggression is as common in psychiatric medicine as it is in marital relationships and it has about it nothing of the appropriate silence in the face of transcendence. Silent aggression is almost always inappropriate and one of the worst of all human coping devices.

The silent doctor can be as cruel and aggressive as the silent patient, and this cruelty may go unnoticed by the doctor. Hippocratic medicine has had a great influence on Western medicine, and silence was advocated by the Hippocratic code of conduct. Science, too, has tended to create the incommunicative doctor, who "doesn't waste time on talk." Then too, there is the problem of malpractice and the ever present danger of something said being used against the doctor later in a lawsuit. All these influences supply a certain justification for silence and hide from the doctor the inappropriateness of this behavior from a human and ethical point of view. For all of these reasons, it is more important from an ethical perspective for doctors to learn to talk than it is to learn to be silent.

Listening is an appropriate form of silence, one that the doctor should develop as part of his character. Silence can be an invitation to relationship, as well as an act of aggression and cruelty. The doctor who listens silently is complimenting the patient and showing interest. Benevolent silence is another way of talking about the kind of listening which creates the condition for the development of a good doctor/patient relationship. Only when the doctor listens well can the patient talk, and patient talk has many benefits. A listening capability is clearly a habit or character trait, and surely one that can be learned.

Truth in Medical Practice

Truthfulness in speech and willingness to talk have not been historical virtues of the physician. The physician Iapix in *The Aeneid* refers to medicine as an *ars muta*, or silent art (*Aen.*, XII, 396-97). In the *Hippocratic corpus*, one finds many references to the practice of not talking to the patient. Writers talked about artful hands and eyes but not of artful words (*Corpus Hippocraticum*—de Arte L.VI, 26, 381). Later on, in *The Laws* (720 and 857), Plato made an explicit distinction between the medicine practiced on slaves which was a *medicina muta*, and the medicine practiced on free men which included talk, and indeed, patient/physician dialogues. The quality of this talk must not have been outstanding because the same Plato, revealing quite a bit about doctors in fourth century Athens, held that lying by physicians was not morally reprehensible. This tradition continues in many cultures. In a recent TV program on medicine in the Soviet Union, a famous Russian doctor proudly pronounced systematic lying to patients in terminal situations as an unalterable standard of Soviet practice.

In most Western democracies, truth has made a comeback in the sense that doctors today consider lying neither to be required in the practice of medicine nor to be justified. Some recent statistical polls reflect this change. Whereas a generation ago, American doctors tended not to tell their patients the truth about dismal prognoses or impending death, now the overwhelming majority of physicians report that they tell the truth even in unpleasant circumstances.[5]

While this change is encouraging, it cannot be interpreted to mean that truthfulness is no longer a problem for American physicians or an issue in bioethics. The basic values on which authentic human life depends are always threatened. Indeed truth has today become so elusive that Pilate's remark suggesting the impossibility of knowing it (What is truth?) is commonly accepted wisdom. Recently, in the course of a conversation with a communist friend, I mentioned that truth has been one of the major casualties in Marxist societies. She just smiled. "And do you think there is any truth in other societies?" she asked.

For American doctors today, the more frequent question is not "What is truth?" but "How do I tell the truth?" "How do I communicate the truth without violating the important obligation of benefiting the patient?" In that sense, truth continues to create difficulties for practicing physicians, and the virtue of truthfulness does not receive the attention it deserves either in clinical training or clinical ethics.

Truthfulness and Benevolence

The virtue of truthfulness refers to a disposition to tell the truth not once, but over and over again. It shows itself in speech and action and in the very being of a person. Truthfulness is, first of all, a foundational element of character, a chosen way of being on the part of the person. Certain habits of truth are learned which express this character trait appropriately in different situations.

All virtues build character, and the special contribution of truthfulness to the inner being of a person is a certain stability, firmness or inner strength. Animals possess this stability by reason of their identification with a stable nature. They are what they are and remain what they are from the beginning to the end of their existence. But man does not possess himself by nature or in a determined way. The inner stability of the human person is an accomplishment rather than a given.

Freely chosen good acts contribute to the development of character, but none contribute to character stability more than truthfulness. Deceit, lying, and all untruthfulness undermine both the stability and the identity of a person. Who is the person who does not tell the truth even to himself? Who knows? If that person is a doctor, can anyone depend on him? Whatever tensions or influences are operating at the moment will dictate what he says and how he acts. On the other hand, when a doctor develops a habit of telling the truth, every truth told confirms and strengthens his inner being. People not only know who he is, but can depend on him. The virtue of truthfulness confirms his character and strengthens his inner being. It constitutes a stable, strong, professional self.

Modern secular persons sometimes smile cynically at any mention of truthfulness because modern society makes truth and truthfulness difficult accomplishments. But still the term "truth" has meaning. And truthfulness means the habit of speaking what one understands to be true. Sometimes, to know what is true is difficult, and sometimes it is difficult even to speak what one knows to be true. But this is not the same as to deny the existence of truth or truthfulness. Even the cynic knows when he is not being truthful: when he is deliberately deceiving someone or hiding the truth or twisting it for convenience. The virtue of truthfulness is a habit of telling the truth even when it is not convenient or does not serve a personal convenience. This virtue rests upon and develops in a person's self the instinctive sense that it is right to be truthful and that truthfulness has to do with the kind of person we come to be.

"Well enough," the doctor may say, "I wish I could tell the truth." "I would prefer to be a truth teller." "I can feel the shrinkage of my character with each lie, and the accumulation of lies at times sickens me." "In some cases, I cannot tell the truth without hurting the patient who asks me for information." "In other cases, I feel obliged to lie because people who have no right to know continually ask me for information." The conflict between doing what is best for the patient and telling the truth to the patient is a real one. But, first we'll look at the issue of lying when persons have no right to know. It is the easiest to dispose of.

All truth telling is predicated upon the assumption that the other person has a right to know the truth. Many of the so-called dilemmas regarding truthfulness found in case books are false dilemmas and, in fact, easily solved. If the inquiring party has no right to know the information which I have, then I have no obligation to communicate it. Without a right to know, there is not a problem of telling the truth, only a problem of avoiding outright untruth. Lying may not be right, but there is nothing at all wrong with avoiding a revelation of information, and prudence will dictate many ways of doing this. One technique commonly used by truthful persons is simply to be silent. We have already spoken of appropriate and inappropriate uses of silence as a type of communication. In some cases silence says, "You have no right to ask that." People get this message and the doctor is not forced to lie. If, in other cases, the doctor is put under intense pressure to reveal something that should not be told, this amounts to violence which causes speech to lose meaning. Sometimes, a doctor may feel morally obliged to guard the truth even at the cost of great personal sacrifice. But that cannot, under all circumstances, be required. Ordinarily, once subjected to violence, doctors (like anyone else) say what they have to say in order to survive. Some deviations or defects do not undermine a person's character the way lying as a matter of habit does.

Situations of violence are rare in modern Western democracies, but an American doctor's commitment to truthfulness may be strained by a conflict with benevolence and the commitment to do what is best for the patient. Every experienced doctor knows that truth is not spoken in a vacuum, but in a clinical context with its own unique characteristics. There is always a particular patient with many different needs other than the need to know the truth. And there is no question here of whether an inquiring party has a right to truth. Now, the issue is how to balance one right with other rights and other duties.

One way of looking at such conflict situations recognizes that truthfulness for the physician must be coordinated with benevolence. The doctor speaks the truth in a moral context dominated by an obligation to do what is best for the patient. Truthfulness ripped out of this context can easily become a wrong and hurtful thing. A context of benevolence means that the emphasis is placed upon when and how and with what sensitivity the truth is communicated to this particular patient with these unique personal needs. Let me provide an example to illustrate this point. A 65-year-old man comes to his physician with complaints of abdominal pain that is persistent, but not extreme. Studies show metastatic cancer of the pancreas. The patient has just retired from a long career and has plans for a 'round-the-world' tour with his wife.[6] There is no doubt that the patient must be told the truth about his condition, but the doctor, in communicating the truth, should take into consideration the patient's particular circumstances and situation. If this context is ignored, truth telling could itself be brutal and possibly harm the patient unnecessarily. There may be times when one can tell the truth without looking left or right, but rarely does the doctor enjoy such a luxury. For the doctor, beneficence considerations are the context in which any question of truthfulness is raised, and physician truth telling can never disregard that context. The doctor's virtue of truthfulness requires both sensitivity and subtlety.

In order that subtleties do not deprive truthfulness of content and character building capabilities, another possibility must be considered. The doctor can become so absorbed by concerns for the patient's welfare that truth disappears as a value and truthfulness with it. Fears for the patient's welfare may literally destroy truthfulness and turn the doctor into a habitual liar. Truth telling in disregard of benevolence can destroy a patient, while an exaggerated benevolent concern for the patient's welfare can erode both truthfulness and the doctor's character.

The virtue of truthfulness, then, stands between these two extremes. Truth must be spoken benevolently, but it must be spoken. When there are concerns about how the truth will affect the patient, the doctor must be aware that truth telling is presumed to be the right thing to do, and that the ethical substance of one's inner self depends upon loyalty to truth. Loyalty to truth is ordinarily the way of benevolence, just as it is the way to a strong, dependable character.

Rather than worrying about whether the truth will hurt the patient, doctors often rightfully worry whether or not what they know is the truth. Is the medical information certain enough to warrant being communicated? Rarely does the doctor's knowledge approach the certainty associated with science—no matter how much modern medicine claims to be an applied science. Scientific laws and reliable predictions just do not operate in human beings as they do in physics. Not only are the variables beyond management, but "unscientific" influences like a positive or negative patient attitude can make all of the difference in a medical outcome. The worst forms of cancer suddenly go into remission and only mild infections sometimes kill. In the face of this uncertainty, the experienced clinician is hesitant to disclose too much either about diagnosis or about prognosis. But here again, benevolence and prudence combine to make possible a truthfulness which is beneficent for the patient without undermining the doctor's character.

The virtue of truthfulness ultimately is important because of its close connection with good doctor/patient relationships. It creates the disposition to acts on which this relationship depends. Truthfulness gives a depth and firmness to the relationship, as well as to the character of the doctor who cultivates and practices it. No relationship can endure failures of truthfulness for long and least of all the doctor/patient relationship. Falsehood destroys community at every level: national, state, business partnerships, parental and marriage relationships, and the doctor/patient relationship. The cultivation of truthfulness is not a fringe issue in medical ethics. It has substantial influence on who the doctor comes to be as a person and what kind of a relationship he develops with his patients.

Conclusion

We can conclude this chapter with a word about the truthfulness that precedes the doctor/patient relationship. Doctors, like other human beings who want to be good, have to struggle to be truthful even with themselves. Not only is the truth about others often hidden below superficial and easily mistaken acts or gestures, but our own inner truth is also hidden from us. The psychiatrist sees self-ignorance and self-deceit frequently in patients, but in mental illness we find them in only the most obvious and extreme cases. Our communication with others requires truth, but so too does our communication with ourselves. Even within ourselves, we are separated into self as known and self as unknown; into viewer and viewed. Consequently, there is a place for the virtue of truthfulness even with ourselves, in the sense of seeing ourselves as we are and admitting to ourselves what we see.

Lying to oneself is just as corrupting as lying in relationships. To lie to oneself is to condemn oneself to self-ignorance, a blight on the inner being of a person either from an ethical or a psychiatric point of view. Great moral philosophers (such as Socrates) and great psychiatric theorists (such as Freud) recognized the corruption of self-deceit and the liberation of self-knowing. For these reasons and for others, doctors who want to be ethical cannot ignore the demands of truthfulness toward themselves. Physicians are vulnerable to self-ignorance and self-deceit because they are persons of power and prestige. People cater to them and infrequently tell them the truth about themselves. As the top authorities in the modern, medical delivery system, doctors usually get their way. They can easily come to think that they are always right and, consequently, ignore their own deep-seated fallibility. It is easier for doctors to see the faults of others than to see their own faults. As a result, it is easy for doctors to develop a narrow and conceited view of themselves, frankly to become fools when it comes to their own inner truth.

But to become a good doctor, one must both know the truth and do the truth. There is no alternative to the struggle to recognize truth and to communicate it in words and actions. The alternative to truthfulness in relationships is to become submerged in deceit and isolated from others. The alternative to truthfulness about one's self is to live in tragic delusion and isolation even from one's self. Given the place of truthfulness in the thousands of ordinary medical acts, doctors who aspire to be good doctors pay attention to this aspect of their character development even though it does not play a very important role in contemporary medical ethics.

Notes

1. The survey was done by Lou Harris and Associates and reported by Victor Cohn in *The Washington Post*. It was also reported in *The Harrisburg Patriot*, Apr. 30, 1985.

2. Another study with similar results was done by Dr. Howard Beckman of Wayne State University Medical School.

3. Lain Entralgo, Pedro, *The Therapy of the Word in Classical Antiquity*. (New Haven: Yale University Press), 1970.

4. Wittgenstein, Ludwig. *Tractatus Logico-Philosophicus*, (New York: Humanities Press), 1961.

5. Novach, Dennis H. et. al., "Changes in Physician's Attitudes Towards Telling the Cancer Patient," *Journal of the American Medical Association*, vol. 241, March, 1979, pp. 897-900.

6. Case used in *Clinical Ethics*, by Jonsen, Siegler, and Winslade, (New York: Macmillan Publishing Co.), 1986, p. 66.

4.

Decision-Making and the Virtue of Respect

Truthful communication between doctor and patient is a good in itself, and the necessary condition for actualizing another basic dimension of the doctor/patient relationship. Patients need to hear the doctor's disclosure and to know the truth about their condition, in order to participate fully in the medical treatment. Besides being cognitive, patients are also autonomous beings. As such, they have a right to decide for themselves what will be done with their bodies. The doctor proposes, but it is the patient of mature years and sound mind who ultimately decides whether any treatment will be started, or if there is more than one medically acceptable option, which one will actually be tried. If the doctor/patient relationship is a communication between two persons, it is also an ethical enterprise, in the sense that both doctor and patient will make free decisions. Benevolence is a virtue which, as we have seen, disposes the doctor to treat his patients in a caring and personal way. Truthfulness disposes the doctor to prepare patients for full participation in decisions regarding their own lives. When patient participation actually occurs, however, the virtue of respect safeguards its integrity.

Truthfulness, as we saw, is the trained disposition to communicate in such a way that the patients understand their situations. Respect is the trained attitude or disposition to reverence those free acts by which patients carry out their best interests. Persons are unique not only in their communication systems, but also because they are endowed with a capacity to choose their own ends and to make their own lives by these choices. This capacity we call freedom or autonomy, and respect is the disposition to reverence this capacity. Respect is to man's capacity for self-determination what truthfulness is to man's capacity for symbolic communication; a virtue which enhances both the other and the one who acts respectfully. Not to respect the patient's freedom is to ignore the reality of the other, to reduce the other to the status of an object, and, indeed, to diminish one's own human status.

What Doctors Choose

To respect the patient is a choice, and respect exercised over and over again creates the virtue of respect. But the doctor makes many other choices which belong to the ethical dimension of the doctor/patient relationship. A simple example will highlight this idea.

Walking down the street, some yards ahead of the doctor, a pedestrian stops, leans against a wall, and then falls unconscious on the sidewalk. The doctor is on his way to the office where patients are already waiting to see him. But rather than looking away and walking by, as several others did, the doctor stops to offer help to the fallen stranger. He turns the person on his back, loosens his collar, checks the vital signs and then asks someone to call an ambulance. If he confirms that the person is not breathing, without hesitation, the doctor begins mouth to mouth resuscitation. When the ambulance arrives, he gives directions to the attendants, and then climbs aboard to accompany the sick person to the hospital.

The very sight of a person fallen ill and in need creates in the doctor a *"ferencia,"* an inclination, a sense of duty to assist (*ad-sistere:* to stand close). Instead of walking by, the doctor elects to stop. Then he chooses to carry out a certain set of technical acts, including mouth to mouth resuscitation. Finally, he decides to stay with the patient, either until the danger is past or until he is able to hand the patient over to specially trained doctors. All of these behaviors are chosen by the doctor and reflect an ethical dimension of the doctor's behavior. In this case, a number of different ethical acts were carried out, but because the patient was critical and incompetent, choosing to respect the patient's freedom means respecting a presumed choice to be treated.

In a less dramatic medical situation, one in which the doctor is seeing a patient who has made an appointment, the doctor chooses to greet the patient in a way which makes him feel accepted and comfortable. Then, she chooses to carry out the diagnosis and treatment in a benevolent and personal way. All the while, there is communication between the two, because the diagnosis is completed only when the doctor provides a clear and personalized explanation to the patient. Finally, we arrive at the focus of this chapter: the choice to respect the patient's decision concerning treatment. Respect for patient choices, however, is part of a larger ethical context, and the virtue of respect which disposes the doctor to reverence the patient must be seen in the context of benevolence and truthfulness rather than as a separate ethical phenomenon.

Precisely because the ethical standards of medicine and their corresponding virtues are rooted in the complexities of the doctor/patient relationship, conflicts sometimes develop among different standards and different virtues. One classic conflict emerges when the doctor feels obliged both to do what is in the patient's best medical interest and also to respect the patient's choice, which may be opposed to that interest. For example, how does the doctor do what is best for the patient in a benevolent and truly personal way, and at the same time, respect what he believes to be the medically detrimental decisions of his patient? We already saw that beneficence is the constitutional principle of medical ethics. The essential medical value is patient welfare. Medicine's golden rule is to do what is in the best interest of the patient or at least not to harm the patient. And benevolence is a virtue disposing the doctor to put this basic principle into practice. As such, benevolence is the ruling virtue, permeating other virtues like truthfulness and, now, the virtue of respect. Of all these virtues, benevolence is the cardinal medical virtue on which the others are hinged. Doctors should cultivate truthfulness, but a truthfulness permeated by benevolence. The same is true of respect for patient autonomy. First, we must see what respect means in itself, and then see how it is coordinated with benevolence in the character of the good physician.

What Respect Means

The English word "respect" derives from the Latin *re-spicere*, which means to look at again, or to look upon, in the sense of giving particular attention and consideration. In a negative sense, respect means not to intrude upon or interfere with another person's privacy. To respect is to recognize the significance of the other and to adopt an appropriate attitude which begins with a stepping back, a refusal to intrude, the keeping of a certain distance. Distance permits the other to be. The more significant the other, the greater the distance and the greater the consideration given.

Keeping distance restrains an inclination to dominate the other, to take possession, or to use the other for one's own ends. Employing a manual analogy, respect is keeping one's hands off, rather than grasping. Respect, then, is a matter of restraint. The virtue of respect disposes a person, first of all, to recognize the significance, dignity, freedom of the other and then to keep enough distance to let the other be. Kant speaks often about respect as the proper response to the essential freedom of the human being in *Lectures on Ethics*[1] and in the first and second parts of *The Metaphysics of Morals.*[2]

Respect is an essential virtue for physicians because it is essential for human development. To exist as human beings, community is necessary, and the most elementary condition for the possibility of community is the disposition of individuals to respect one another as free and self-determining. Children need respect as much as the elderly and, so too, do persons at all the intermediate stages. Respect makes possible association rather than combat and is intimately linked with other basic values like benevolence, kindness, justice, etc. Ethics for physicians begins, like any humanistic ethics, with a recognition of the value and dignity of human persons.

Since the doctor/patient relationship, like any other, involves free and independent persons with different interests, ends and goals, strains will develop. The patient's lifestyle, value system, and way of being will often be very different from the doctor's. Consequently, what the doctor believes is best for the patient may not at all agree with the patient's conviction about his or her own welfare. Respect is the virtue which disposes the doctor to handle such differences with sensitivity, avoiding either deceit or manipulation. Manipulation, deceit and fraud are intrusions into the very inner being of the other person and a violation of the distance essential for respect.

When respect is talked about in contemporary bio-ethics, it usually means respect for privacy. So many aspects of life, today, are talked about as privacy matters that the referent of the word "privacy" has become diffuse and its meaning confused. (For example, some of the most blatant forms of public behavior are called private matters.) Suppose we happen to see a child with hands folded and eyes closed, totally absorbed in prayer. Obviously, what is going on here is private. Respect for privacy means not to interfere, not to make the child a spectacle, not to use the child's intimate communication for some selfish gain. A woman who has just learned that her beloved husband was killed in an accident and who is sobbing in distress, just as obviously, is engaged in a private matter which warrants maintaining a sensitive distance. In both cases, the person's inner being is manifest in physical behaviors, and this makes it easier to understand what respect for privacy requires. Not every feeling, belief, decision of a person is so impressively reflected in visible form or imposes an almost instinctual respect, and yet human feelings, beliefs and decisions belong to the inner being of the public person and, therefore, call for the same respect of privacy.

Respect is elemental in real life, as well as in Kant's moral theory, because it is derived from the very structure of persons and relationships. Where it is missing or insufficiently developed, both persons and relationships fail. Friendships fail when one friend loses respect for the other or uses the other for gain.[3] Kant again spells out this connection in the chapter on "friendship" in his *Lectures on Ethics*. The same is true of marriages. If one partner does not feel respected, then insecurity mounts and intimacy diminishes. Without respect, there can be no intimacy and, therefore, love declines. Estranged partners almost always talk of being treated as objects rather than persons. And what is true of friendship and marriage is true of the doctor/patient relationship. Its very structure requires respect, just as it requires benevolence and truthfulness on the part of the doctor. The true friend, the successful spouse, and the good doctor have all developed the virtue of respect. But respect in the doctor/patient relationship has some special features.

Patients of doctors who are well known find themselves confronted with a certain greatness. Distinguished doctors qualify for greatness because of the demands they have placed upon themselves. Their efforts, as well as their originality, creativity, boldness of decision, breadth of understanding and depth of commitment to their profession stand out above the rest. The proper response to such greatness on the part of the patient is a certain distance and respect. Without respect, anger and resentment quickly develop. Instead of rejoicing in the doctor's greatness, nonrespectful patients look for ways of destroying what causes them discomfort. They look for faults, criticize and generally try to reduce the doctor's stature. Respect, on the other hand, lets the greatness of the other be. It provides space even for greater persons, although "I am not great." Respect as a virtue is the only alternative to envy and resentment, which are destructive of both self and others. The person who respects distinction, however, is able to stand alongside greatness and thereby enjoy its benefits. The structural unevenness of the doctor/patient relationship makes some degree of "greater and lesser" inevitable.

The doctor's respect is grounded in an appropriate awe before each unique patient. For him, respect is based not so much upon what a patient may or may not have done, but who the person is. Excellence of accomplishments deserves recognition, but so too does excellence of being. One of the dangers to which the modern physician is exposed is to lose sight of this when the being of the patient is reduced to a number in a long line or a complex of purely physical responses. Once the doctor thinks of himself consciously or unconsciously as an engineer working on a piece of machinery rather than in relationship with other persons, the ground of respect is lost. Just because the engineering model is so powerful in this age of technological medicine, an emphasis is needed on the patient as person. Effort is required by the doctor to develop the virtue of respect precisely because the medical environment today tends to form the doctor in the opposite direction. And yet, without reverence and respect, even a technically accomplished physician cannot be a good doctor.

To be a good doctor, a physician has to be different. For many people in competitive secular cultures, weakness and defensiveness are invitations to exploitation. For the good doctor, just the opposite is the case. The good doctor helps, talks to and respects those who are weak and defenseless. Patients invite from the good doctor a response similar to what children invite from adults who have normal moral development. Only the morally perverse violate children, and only morally flawed doctors do not respect patients. The virtue of respect is not a frill, but rather an essential dimension of any medical ethics which addresses common, everyday medical acts and not just unusual cases.

How Respect for Autonomy Functions in Medicine

Usually what the doctor believes to be best for the patient will also be what the patient freely determines to be in his own best interest. But both goods, the good of the patient's welfare from the medical point of view and the good from the patient's own personal perspective, are not always smoothly integrated. What happens when the two goods are opposed rather than synthesized? Does the doctor give more weight and importance to the objective medical values of curing, relieving pain and restoring function, or to subjective values which perhaps stand behind a patient's rejection of medical help? Obviously, both are important, and a proper balancing is called for. But how can the doctor justify deference to patient preferences? At some point, doing what the patient prefers may mean violating the constitutional principle and cardinal virtue of medicine. At some point, respecting the patient's wishes may mean not practicing good medicine. Some light may be shed on this dilemma by looking at another profession.

A democratic culture finds it necessary to put up with all sorts of bad taste, untruths and injustices so as not to undermine freedom, the essential ethical value of the profession of journalism. Rather than interfere with freedom of the press, all sorts of bad press is put up with, along with its bad influence on society. Freedom is so important for the exercise of journalism in democracy that disvalues are tolerated, in order to protect the essential value of freedom. By analogy, beneficence (and benevolence) is to medicine what freedom is to journalism. Certainly, other values are involved in medicine as they are in journalism, and ideally all values are realized. But in the case of conflict, the essential value must prevail. Doctors cannot be turned into promoters of patient freedom anymore than journalists can be turned into promoters of some vision of social justice or social welfare. The essential and characteristic values of key professions must be protected by law, even if other important values have to take second place or be limited. Medicine is a key profession in society, and citizen health a basic societal concern.

Obviously, this does not mean that doctors can simply do what they think best or ignore the patient's wishes. The power of the doctor today is considerable, and it must be used, as we have seen all along, in the most humane way. Doctors cannot simply do what they think is best because this would convert the patient into a thing and violate medicine's essential value. Medical ethics requires that doctors do what is in the patient's best medical interest in a human way. This final prepositional phrase creates real limits to the exercise of beneficence. Doctors can (power) always do more than they ought (ethics), and therefore limits to physician power are crucial. But doctors cannot be forced to violate their essential and constitutional principle.

Doing what will most benefit the patient medically is the doctor's primary ethical responsibility. This he or she must do competently, benevolently and truthfully. Now we must add another adverb: respectfully. This means that the competent and careful doctor, who has every right to be respected himself in what pertains to his medical judgments, must respect the personal preferences of the patient. The patient's welfare cannot be reduced simply to what is in the patient's best medical interests. Patient personal interests and beliefs make up an important part of what is medically beneficial. Doing what is medically best for the patient or promoting a patient's best medical interest requires that the patient's own beliefs about what is medically best be taken into consideration and respected. But beneficence remains the primary principle and benevolence, the cardinal virtue in medical ethics.

In order that medical best interests not be subordinated to the other values, medical codes and hospital policies should make clear the place these values have in medical practice. Everyone agrees that the state should never be permitted to require doctors to do what may be in the state's best interest but not in the patient's best medical interest. This would undermine the moral foundation of medicine and turn doctors into state functionaries. The same is true for insurance companies, hospital administrations, and HMO directors. The physician's essential ethical value cannot be permitted to be undermined in the interest even of other important values, like autonomy. If doctors must respect patients, the same respect must be shown to doctors by patients. Doctors cannot be obligated to do what they do not believe to be beneficial or what they believe to be maleficent. Bio-ethicists who think of the doctor/patient relationship as a purchase of services in which the consumer (the patient) is in full control do not consider what being ill is all about and the importance of medicine as a profession to society. If journalism is important, so too is medicine, and each profession has its own ethical foundation and its own basic ethical principle which must be safeguarded.

The Delicate Balance

A balancing of values in conflict situations is part of medical ethics, and this implies that the weight will come down differently in different situations. As a patient slips ever further from the doctor's power to benefit, then strictly objective medical values give way to non-medical ones. For a doctor to continue to insist strictly on what would be best from a medical perspective, as a patient moves toward death, is equivalent to condemning every patient to a medical rather than a personal death. Here, better than anywhere, we can see the need for keeping different values and virtues in balance. As the patient moves from an acute and easily cured illness into chronic illness and finally into greatly reduced quality of life and the dying process, beneficence, as medical best interest weighs less, and autonomy, as patient personal preference, weighs more. Doctors who are respectful recognize this value shift and make appropriate adjustments.

But every patient interest, need, belief and decision cannot be respected if medicine is to retain its self-esteem and to serve society. Limits on what doctors can respect in patient preferences and decisions come from standards of good medical practice, the effect of the patient's decision on others, and the interest of the state. Some decisions are strictly medical ones, and patients have no right to intervene in these (e.g., choosing an antibiotic). Others are strictly personal, in the face of which the physician's only moral attitude has to be respect (e.g. whether to have tubes tied to limit family size). And still others depend upon both (e.g., which medical option to use in the case of breast cancer). In every medical situation, more than one value is involved, and, more than one virtue is called for.

As crucial as the principle of beneficence is to the integrity of medicine and the virtue of benevolence to the ethics of a practicing physician, other principles and virtues also figure in an adequate medical ethics. The good doctor must also be disposed to communicate with the patient about health issues and then to develop attitudes of respect for the patient's participation in decisions about what is to be done. The virtue of respect protects the patient against domination by increasing sensitivity for the patient's interests and needs. Besides contributing substantially to the character of the doctor, it permits patients to make decisions which reflect their own character and values, as well as satisfies and important patient need.

The virtue of respect shows itself concretely in the doctor's attention to all the legal and ethical elements of a truly informed consent. Much of the animosity people feel toward doctors derives from actual experiences of a loss of control in the medical setting or from fears that hospitalization will mean loss of power over their own lives. For weak, partially incompetent, seriously ill elderly persons, for example, this fear is realistic. Studies of patient uncooperativeness in hospitals show how often it results from not having been shown the minimal signs of respect. Patients want to be talked to and consulted with about what is being done to them. Despite so much talk about patient rights and medical ethics, patients in high-tech, acute care facilities frequently have the feeling of being treated as things in an industrial process. All the treatises on informed consent, and all the court cases defining its constituent elements, have not changed the depersonalizing experience of hospital patients. Developing a virtue of respect for patient decisions also flies in the face of a 2,500 year old tradition which respected patients as parents respect children but not as adults respect other adults.

Notes

1. Kant, Immanuel. *Lectures on Ethics*, Harper Torch Books, (New York: Harper Torch Books, Harper and Row), 1963. Chapters on "Proper Self-Respect" and "Duties Toward Others."

2. Kant, Immanuel. *The Metaphysical Principles of Virtue*, Part Two of *The Metaphysics of Morals*, James Ellington, trns., (New York: Bobbs Merrill Co.), 1964.

3. Kant again spells out this connection in the chapter on "Friendship" in his *Lectures on Ethics.*

5.

Inevitability of Feelings and the Virtue of Friendliness

Whenever we meet other persons, we look at them and are immediately aware either of a pleasant or unpleasant feeling associated with the encounter. In popular language, talk of good or bad chemistry refers to this immediate feeling dimension of human meetings. Among the many components which together constitute the complex human relationship is an affective one. People who meet, feel something for one another: either an affection or an antipathy. Relationship involves knowing, acting, communicating, choosing and also feeling. There is a cognitive, operative, communicative, ethical and now an affective dimension to the coming together of persons.

What is true of relationships in general, is also true of the specific doctor/patient relationship. From the very moment in which doctor and patient meet, they express in different internal and external acts all the dimensions of a human meeting. Doctors, like everyone else, are affected by other people. Besides knowing and acting and talking and choosing, doctors inevitably feel something toward patients and patients do the same. In this chapter, we want to look at the affect produced both in the doctor and in the patient by a medical encounter, as well as those attitudes and dispositions of the inner self (virtues) which promote the right kind of affect. At the very beginning, however, a disclaimer is needed. Despite its importance in medicine, affection does not develop in absolutely every doctor/patient encounter.

Although affect usually develops in a doctor/patient relationship, there are medical situations in which it simply does not happen. If the doctor is a surgeon and is called to perform an emergency operation on an unconscious accident victim, some slight affect may develop as the doctor reviews the patient's present status and personal background, but not much. And certainly, the patient cannot feel much toward the doctor. And there are many other examples of this same phenomenon. If a patient happens to be particularly reserved, a thoroughly inner-directed type of personality, and is visiting a company doctor for an annual check-up, there may be some feeling dimension to this relationship, but not much. Finally, if the patient happens to find himself in a large, university medical center, where medical care is carried out by teams, the opportunities for affect to develop in the doctor/patient relationship are very limited.

Without doubt, contemporary medical practice puts severe negative pressures on the affective dimension of the doctor/patient relationship, but rarely do the objectifying influences completely extinguish this characteristically human dimension in the medical encounter. Given half a chance, doctors and patients develop feelings for one another. Precisely because of the many negative pressures upon the development of affection, however, more attention needs to be paid to this dimension, and to the virtue which disposes the doctor toward proper feelings for his patient.

Freud was the first to articulate a detailed theoretical explanation of the feelings which develop between doctor and patient, but he was not the first to recognize either the existence or the importance of affection in the medical relationship. The Hippocratic Code and writings had a great deal to say about philanthropy, a form of love not much appreciated today but unmistakeably a form of affection. Paracelsus, in a beautiful statement about the place of affect in the doctor/patient relationship said, "The very deepest foundation of medicine is love... If our love is great, the fruits derived from it in medicine will also be great; and if it is weak, the medical fruits too will be weak. It is love that leads us to learn the medical art and without love, no one becomes a real physician."[1]

The notion that love of a special medical sort is the proper bond between doctor and patient continued through the centuries in Christian culture. After suffering something of a decline with the advent of science and technology, this traditional ideal is making something of a comeback. All the talk about the place of humanities in medicine reflects a resurgence of belief that the best medicine is personalized medicine, medicine in which there is real affect in the relationship between doctor and patient.

People who think about their experience, either as doctors or patients, recognize that there is definitely a feeling tone to the doctor-patient relationship. Most patients have strong positive feelings for their doctors, and where this is not the case, the intensity of the negative feeling reminds us of how people react to disappointed love. There are many reasons why doctors are more vulnerable than any other professionals to lawsuits, but one reason certainly has to do with the strong affect which is part of the doctor/patient relationship and the potential for "getting back" when this affect turns sour. On the side of the doctor, there are also feelings and, although usually they are not as intense as the feelings of the patient, they frequently become intense. Doctors tend to develop either very positive or very negative feelings for their patients.

The Transference

With his first famous psychiatric patient, Sigmund Freud was confronted with the peculiar love which Anna O. developed for her doctor. Breuer, who treated Anna, first fled from her and from the practice of the emerging specialty of psychoanalysis. Freud, on the other hand, joined a puritanical moral rigor with a strong scientific curiosity and was able to understand in depth the unusual feeling dimension of the doctor/patient relationship without being overwhelmed by personal involvement. In fact, for Freud the affective dimension, which he called "transference," became the focus of his therapeutic intervention.

Freud's ideas about affect in medicine were developed from reflection on the doctor/patient relationship in psychoanalysis, but they apply at least to some degree in many other doctor/patient contacts. Freud recognized this. In his mature works, he held that the transference is a dimension of every medical relationship, and the success of the doctor's interventions depend upon an understanding of this factor. One can find a preview of this idea as early as 1895, in Freud's *Studies on Hysteria*. In that book, he held that a personal relationship inevitably develops between the doctor and the patient and that this relationship has a distinct affective tone.[2]

Any time contact between doctor and patient goes on for some time and treatment requires a close collaboration, the affective dimension makes itself too obvious to miss. Ordinarily, the interest and sympathy which the doctor shows for the patient, joined to the esteem which the doctor enjoys, are enough to generate strong positive feelings on the part of the patient. Correspondingly, when neither interest nor sympathy is shown, resulting in the absence of esteem, strong negative feelings develop toward the doctor. Doctors help their patients, answer their questions, provide counsel, even function in many cases as a confessor to whom secret thoughts and actions are revealed. How could strong feelings help but develop in the midst of such intimacy?

Freud thought that the origins of these feelings were to be found in the patient's childhood. In time of need and helplessness, patients undergo a natural, psychological regression. Sickness creates the need for a parent who will care and protect, and the doctor is expected to satisfy this need. Unconsciously (in most cases), patients not only expect parental behavior from doctors, but "transfer" to the doctor feelings that they once had for their parents. This phenomenon explains not just the strong positive affection which patients have for a trusted doctor, but also the bitter disappointment some feel when the doctors do not respond in a properly affectionate way. The intense hostility which some patients have for physicians (without foundation or factual mistreatment) may be explained by negative feelings they harbor toward parents or parental figures. Obviously, there is an affective dimension to the doctor/patient relationship, and, just as obviously, doctors need to be aware of it and to develop habits of appropriate response.

Because of pressures deriving from technology and impersonal institutions, the natural affection between doctor and patient sometimes either does not develop or develops but nowhere near as strongly as with Freud's patients. In certain cases, a doctor can accurately diagnose and effectively treat without developing any personal relationship, let alone affection for the patient. In other cases, personal contact and an affective dimension develop in the relationship, but both are transitory and superficial. Finally, some patients have reduced capacities for relationships of any sort, and others consider doctors to be technicians unworthy of the effort required to establish a personal relationship.

Despite all this, rarely will the contact between doctor and patient slip to the level of the contact between an airline employee at the ticket counter and a passenger, a purely external and formal friendliness. The airline employee may treat the passenger in what appears to be a warm, friendly way, but if there is any authenticity at all to the affection, it lasts only until the transaction is finished. The same employee in the airport bar or restaurant just a few minutes later will probably neither recognize nor speak to the passenger. At the very least, doctor and patient do better than that. The requirements of diagnosis, the seriousness of illness, and the length of the treatment will all have an impact on the depth of the relationship, but usually a real affective relationship does develop. Doctors will recognize their patient days or weeks after their meeting.

A low level, but real affection, could be compared with what develops between comrades who share political ideals and work for the same political goals. Another metaphor may come from economics. People who work for the same company or collaborate on business projects usually develop a certain level of affection for one another. In ordinary language, we talk about "friends from work" to distinguish them from deeper forms of friendship. Doctors and patients may become "friends" for awhile, at least while they work together on a project of the patient's health. Such collaboration involves relationship and a level of affection, although it does not approach the intensity of "transference" and remains far from what we call love.

Friendship

The classical texts talked most often about love between the doctor and the patient, but today a more appropriate term seems to be "friendship." Friendship is love, but without the erotic connotations of "transference" or the religious dimensions of "agape." In his classical text, *De Beneficiis* (VI 16), Seneca wrote about friendship between himself and his doctor.

"Why is it that I owe something more to my physician and my teacher, and yet do not complete the payment of what is due to them? Because from being physician and teacher they pass into friends, and we are under obligation to them, not because of their skill, which they sell, but because of their kindly and friendly goodwill. If, therefore, a physician does nothing more than feel my pulse, and put me on the list of those whom he visits in his rounds, instructing me what to do or what to avoid, but without any personal feeling, I owe him nothing more than his fee, because he views me, not as a friend, but as a commander. (Seneca means, one who demands his professional service.) Nor is there any reason why I should venerate a teacher if he has considered me merely one of his many pupils, and has not deemed me worthy of any particular and special consideration, if he has not directed his attention to me, but has allowed me, not so much to learn from him as to pick up any knowledge that he spilled into our midst. What reason, then, do we have for being much indebted to them? It is not that what they have sold is worth more than we paid for it, but that they have contributed something to us personally. Suppose a physician gave me more attention than was professionally necessary; that it was not for his professional reputation, but for me, that he feared; that he was not content to indicate remedies, but also applied them; that he sat at my bedside among my anxious friends, that he hurried to me at the crises of my illness; that no service was too burdensome, none too distasteful for him to perform; that he was not indifferent when he heard my moans; that, though a host of others called for him, I was always his chief concern; that he took time for others only when my illness permitted him—such a man has placed me under obligation, not as a physician, but as a friend.[3]

In a very contemporary fashion, Seneca distinguishes friendship from the lesser relationship doctors usually have with patients. The doctor may be proper and technically competent, yet he may not establish a personal bond or affection. The affective bond between Seneca and his doctor derived from the doctor's personal interest in holding Seneca's welfare above his own, in personal attention to the administrations of therapy, in being solicitous and in undertaking difficult therapeutic tasks without complaint. Seneca said that his pains affected his doctor, causing him to feel and share the agony. For all these reasons, Seneca thought of his doctor affectionately as a friend, but primarily, because of all the doctor's patients, Seneca felt that he was his doctor's main preoccupation. One could hardly improve on Seneca's text for understanding ideally what affection between doctor and patient means and the enormous positive effect it has on the patient. In holding friendship as the ideal in the doctor/patient relationship, Seneca followed no less an authority than Plato, himself, who talked in the *Lysis* (217 a) about the patient being a friend of his doctor because of his illness.

What Plato and Seneca say about friendship in medicine remains both an ideal and an obligation even for a modern physician. A physician's obligations are still grounded on and derived from the patient's need. We have seen that each dimension of the doctor/patient relationship is influenced by the basic medical principle of beneficence and each virtue is influenced by benevolence. When we speak of the affective dimension and of friendship, therefore, we are talking about affect which develops between a particular patient and this particular physician who offers help. The affect is personal and is intimately related to all the ways a doctor of "good (*bene*) will (*volence*)" treats his patient. It is not, therefore, by chance that all the ways in which Seneca's doctor showed love happened to coincide with what we might describe as benevolence. Benevolence, as we saw, refers primarily to the will to help. Friendship refers primarily to the affective tone of the benevolence, but both virtues arise out of the structure of the doctor/patient relationship and from the patient's needs.

Friendship—And the Meaning of Illness

The patient's need for diagnosis, treatment, communication and participation in decision-making are obvious enough, but does the patient really need love in the form of friendship? Even if affect inevitably develops in the patient for all the reasons Freud alluded to, can we say that patients "need" affection in the same way they need diagnosis and therapy, communication and freedom to choose? Would it not be better simply to note this aspect of the doctor/patient relationship, but not include it with the others or try to argue that doctors have an obligation to develop friendly dispositions? Does the patient really need affection? Does the doctor's affect really help? To some extent, the answer depends upon the type of patient and the degree of illness.

What Freud found in his patients continues to develop today, especially in the chronically and acutely ill. Regression in these situations is altogether natural and creates a strong need for parent-like help. Such patients want and need to be cared for by a doctor who, besides being competent, shows affection, much like that which they received from parents when they were ill. Affection is not just a need and a strong expectation, but an important element in effective therapy.

The character traits of a good doctor are related to patient needs which, in turn, derive from what it means to be ill. Illness moves people to search out a physician who will help them. Some aspects of illness are well known, but others escape all but a close and careful observer. Illness is differently defined in the history of medicine, accordingly as different paradigms are used to understand it, but behind the shifts in theoretical constructs and corresponding conceptual categories, there is a lived reality which people of different ages and cultures refer to as being ill.

Lived experience of illness usually involves a greater or lesser dysfunction. Ill persons cannot carry out some of the functions which are commonly considered a normal part of life. The body permits us to be in the world, and to do certain things, but when illness comes, the "I can do" dimension of physical life is reduced. To a greater or lesser extent, illness means "I can't do." I can't run, or remember, or work, or play. The very words for illness (dis-ease, in-firmity) reflect this experience. And we know, too, that illness implies the opposite of well-being and frequently is associated with feelings of depression, anxiety, antipathy, despair and pain. The body of the ill person which before was silent now speaks in unpleasant tones. The body which before was hardly noticed and made it possible for me to do everything I wanted to do suddenly becomes a heavy weight. I become alienated from my body when I am ill; my body rebels against me and inflicts pain on me. All these experiences are fairly common and well known.

But we may not be as aware of the element of threat in illness. We tend to forget about the risk involved in being a human being, but illness forces the reality of threat back into our consciousness. Illness reminds us of the transitory character of life, and the experience of illness is threatening because it reminds us of death. All of a sudden, certain projects that make me the person I am are in danger of never being realized, and therefore, my very life is in danger of not being fulfilled. Illness brings threats both of a physical and psychological sort, and it is no wonder that illness causes even mature persons to regress a little, to look for protection, to look for someone who will stand by and show affection.

Illness also causes isolation. It makes a person feel alone. My pains are mine and cannot be communicated. Illness forces me to live in them alone. Sometimes there is a social isolation which accompanies the psychological one. Besides the isolation of absorption in one's own discomfort, there is the physical separation from other human beings and normal activities. The isolation is intensified if the ill person is transferred to a hospital room; a kind of solitary confinement broken only partially during fixed visiting hours. It may sound strange, but the truth is that sick persons are ambivalent about visitors. In one sense, they provide a welcome break from the confinement; in another sense, they are a special form of suffering.

Well people cannot really relieve the isolation of persons who are ill; only doctors can. People who are well, happy, strong and enjoying life make the ill person even more aware of pain and isolation. Some cultures isolate the sick more than we do, even ritually excommunicating them from the community. This may not be as cruel as it first appears. At very least, it makes this point in a forceful way: illness involves an isolation which only the doctor can relieve. The seriously ill person is separated from others and forced to abide in his own uncommunicable misery. Every human being needs another who can share experiences, and that other person for a patient is the doctor. The affective dimension of the doctor/patient relationship is not a fringe phenomenon. It is an essential component of a medical relationship. Because of the nature of illness, patients really need affection from a friend who can share what they are suffering and can offer some ray of hope for relief. Patients need a medical friend.

Medical Friendship

The affective dimension of the doctor/patient relationship has all the generic notes of an ordinary friendship: there is pleasure in one another's company, confidences are shared, and there is an exchange of benefits.

For all the reasons alluded to above, patients like the doctor's company and like to be visited by the doctor. If doctors only realized what their visit means, they would not be so anxious to get it over with. For patients, the doctor's visit is the visit of a needed friend. No one else can meet the patient's need. When the pleasure of a doctor's company is denied because of a rushed schedule, patients are disappointed and frequently angry. "Not spending enough time with me" is one of the most frequently heard complaints of patients. Oddly enough, doctors are also depriving themselves. They could enjoy really good feelings from their patients, if only they gave themselves enough time to savor being together. The affection patients bring to the medical encounter obviously has great potential benefit for the physician. Good doctors are aware of the affection and love they receive from their patient-friends.

In medical friendship, feelings are shared and intimacies revealed appropriate only within this relationship. The ancient obligation of secrecy has its roots in friendship; violations of confidentiality are violations of friendship. The patient friend not only has a "feeling of confidence" in the doctor, but "shares many confidences" with him or her. Friends tell each other things no one else has been told. This sharing is part of the bond of friendship and an expression of that bond. What is said in the doctor/patient relationship has all the marks of what is said among friends. It is a somewhat one-sided and unequal sharing because the doctor does not talk about himself or reveal personal intimacies, but what he says to the patient about the patient's illness has a confidential character. Confidentiality means that "What I know about you, I will reveal only to you or to others only with your permission." It makes no sense independent of friendship.

Finally, friends do things for one another.
why his doctor was a friend, he listed his ma
done for one another in the medical relation
with curing and helping. Beneficence and
benevolence are the cardinal moral values in
to the most important medical acts. Friends
a dimension of benevolence. Seneca gave a
tor was a friend, and the reasons all had to d

But for Seneca, the final and most forc
the sense he had of being his doctor's first
that there are other relationships, but the
comes first. Feelings of affection, love, an
in response to the attentions which the doc
that "I am the first preoccupation" or "I an
terests and efforts" naturally gives rise to a
natural response to what the doctor does fo

But does the patient do anything for
benefits which the doctor derives? At first
The patient is looking for help from the
the inevitable inequality of the doctor/pati
more closely, the patient who is helped ac
Not only does the doctor receive affectio
is helped by patients from whom he learn
professional satisfaction.

For all the above reasons, one can ta
the doctor/patient relationship that jus
friendship. Between one person in need
sonalized way, there is frequently an a
components of true friendship. Even wh
realized, a disposition to be friendly and
sential ethical form to everyday doctor/p

From the doctor's side, for example, too mu
make for a lack of affection. On the patient's
equal rights, suspicion or unresolved conflict
the same effect.

At the other end of the spectrum are peculi
excess affection. Doctors, as well as patients
tionate, and friendship can spill into an eroti
patients are more prone to fall in love with t
women with their male gynecologists: w
psychiatrist of the opposite sex. The length of ti
and the level of intimacy involved in the treatme
tribute to the possibility of affection leading
sexual involvements. Sexual contact with psych
wrong if for no other reason than it is destructiv
sive affection, however, in any doctor/patient
pected to diminish therapeutic possibilities, an
violation of professional conduct.

Not quite so obvious are failures of friend
Freud called "negative transference" and "coun
Sometimes the doctor/patient relationship is full
beginning. If the doctor is unfamiliar with Fre
unprovoked hostilities develop in the medical re
possible to work through this problem effectively
may be expressing a forgotten or unforgotten hos
the same sex as the doctor. And the doctor's
colored by early childhood feelings. What F
counter transference can help doctors keep their
under control, and keep the worse type failures o
ring. For the positive promotion of the medical f
doctor needs to give attention and exert effort i
virtue of friendliness.

Medical Friendship

The affective dimension of the doctor/patient relationship has all the generic notes of an ordinary friendship: there is pleasure in one another's company, confidences are shared, and there is an exchange of benefits.

For all the reasons alluded to above, patients like the doctor's company and like to be visited by the doctor. If doctors only realized what their visit means, they would not be so anxious to get it over with. For patients, the doctor's visit is the visit of a needed friend. No one else can meet the patient's need. When the pleasure of a doctor's company is denied because of a rushed schedule, patients are disappointed and frequently angry. "Not spending enough time with me" is one of the most frequently heard complaints of patients. Oddly enough, doctors are also depriving themselves. They could enjoy really good feelings from their patients, if only they gave themselves enough time to savor being together. The affection patients bring to the medical encounter obviously has great potential benefit for the physician. Good doctors are aware of the affection and love they receive from their patient-friends.

In medical friendship, feelings are shared and intimacies revealed appropriate only within this relationship. The ancient obligation of secrecy has its roots in friendship; violations of confidentiality are violations of friendship. The patient friend not only has a "feeling of confidence" in the doctor, but "shares many confidences" with him or her. Friends tell each other things no one else has been told. This sharing is part of the bond of friendship and an expression of that bond. What is said in the doctor/patient relationship has all the marks of what is said among friends. It is a somewhat one-sided and unequal sharing because the doctor does not talk about himself or reveal personal intimacies, but what he says to the patient about the patient's illness has a confidential character. Confidentiality means that "What I know about you, I will reveal only to you or to others only with your permission." It makes no sense independent of friendship.

Finally, friends do things for one another. When Seneca talked about why his doctor was a friend, he listed his many medical acts. The things done for one another in the medical relationship are things having to do with curing and helping. Beneficence and the corresponding virtue of benevolence are the cardinal moral values in medicine because they refer to the most important medical acts. Friendship, like the other virtues, is a dimension of benevolence. Seneca gave a list of reasons why his doctor was a friend, and the reasons all had to do with medical help.

But for Seneca, the final and most forceful proof of friendship was the sense he had of being his doctor's first preoccupation. Friends know that there are other relationships, but the friend knows that he or she comes first. Feelings of affection, love, and friendship arise in patients in response to the attentions which the doctor directs to them. The sense that "I am the first preoccupation" or "I am the center of the doctor's interests and efforts" naturally gives rise to affection which is the patient's natural response to what the doctor does for him.

But does the patient do anything for the doctor? Are there any benefits which the doctor derives? At first, the answer seems to be "no." The patient is looking for help from the doctor, and that is the basis of the inevitable inequality of the doctor/patient relationship. But looked at more closely, the patient who is helped actually provides many benefits. Not only does the doctor receive affection and confidences, but he also is helped by patients from whom he learns and through whom he derives professional satisfaction.

For all the above reasons, one can talk of an affective dimension to the doctor/patient relationship that justifies being called a medical friendship. Between one person in need and another who helps in a personalized way, there is frequently an affection which satisfies all the components of true friendship. Even when full blown friendship is not realized, a disposition to be friendly and a will to friendship gives an essential ethical form to everyday doctor/patient contacts.

Managing the Dangers of an Affective Relationship

Medical friendship has both peculiarities and peculiar problems. Doctors hold preeminence over patients because of the power they wield. An "ideally equal" relationship simply does not work in medicine because the doctor is more powerful and because the patient's belief and trust in the doctor's superior power is an important dimension of theraputic effectiveness. To insist on equality in medicine is like insisting on equality in the teacher/student relationship. The two are not equal, and attempts to force an equality destroy both the teacher's function and the benefits she may bring to the student. The same is true of the doctor. The power which the doctor wields is differently understood by different patients. Modern educated people tend to understand the doctor's power in rationalistic terms; that is, superior knowledge. Less academically oriented persons may interpret a doctor's power straightforwardly in terms of authority: the power of a mother or a father. Others adopt what we could call a religious view of the doctor and see his or her power as a type of magic. More often than not, the patient's interpretation of the doctor's power and preeminence turns out to be a combination of all the above. There is neither reason to change nor any way to change the essential inequality of the doctor/patient relationship, and yet, as we have seen, the weaker partner is a human person with all the respect due any and all persons. Therefore, peculiar as it may sound, the medical relationship is at the same time, equal and unequal. But this is not the only peculiarity.

Some of the problems peculiar to the affective dimension of the doctor/patient relationship can easily be imagined, but not all. Some doctors, simply stated, are cold and unfriendly and undisposed to affection of any sort, let alone to friendship. The causes of the coldness are many: a cold personality, dislike for the work, a belief that aloofness is the scientifically required posture of a good doctor, to mention only a few. And what is true of doctors is true, as well, of patients. Either from one side or the other, there can be coldness and lack of capacity for affection.

From the doctor's side, for example, too much interest in money can make for a lack of affection. On the patient's side, an overconcern with equal rights, suspicion or unresolved conflict with parents has exactly the same effect.

At the other end of the spectrum are peculiar problems coming from excess affection. Doctors, as well as patients, can become too affectionate, and friendship can spill into an erotic involvement. Certain patients are more prone to fall in love with their doctors than others: women with their male gynecologists: women and men with a psychiatrist of the opposite sex. The length of time spent with the doctor and the level of intimacy involved in the treatment process certainly contribute to the possibility of affection leading to mutual seduction and sexual involvements. Sexual contact with psychiatric patients is morally wrong if for no other reason than it is destructive of the therapy. Excessive affection, however, in any doctor/patient relationship, can be expected to diminish therapeutic possibilities, and therefore represents a violation of professional conduct.

Not quite so obvious are failures of friendship from defect: what Freud called "negative transference" and "counter transference upsets." Sometimes the doctor/patient relationship is full of hostilty from the very beginning. If the doctor is unfamiliar with Freud's explanation of how unprovoked hostilities develop in the medical relationship, it will be impossible to work through this problem effectively. The patient, in reality, may be expressing a forgotten or unforgotten hostility toward a parent of the same sex as the doctor. And the doctor's reaction may also be colored by early childhood feelings. What Freud has to say about counter transference can help doctors keep their own negative responses under control, and keep the worse type failures of friendship from occurring. For the positive promotion of the medical friendship, however, the doctor needs to give attention and exert effort in the cultivation of the virtue of friendliness.

The Virtue of Friendliness

Everyone recognizes the need human beings have for friends. Absence of friends can bring a young person to the point of suicide. Finding a friend, on the other hand, can turn everything around. Young people talk more about friends, but friends are crucial at every age. The Greek philosophers included friends among the most precious of human goods, but not much attention is given either in classical or modern literature to the traits which help a person to develop friends. Perhaps friendliness is thought to be solely a matter of natural disposition and having good friends strictly a matter of luck, but this view is simplistic. Some people slip into unfriendly ways and others work successfully to develop friendliness. Obviously, it helps a great deal to have a naturally friendly disposition, but virtues are cultivated as well as natural. Although not much attention is paid to it in American culture, there is such a thing as moral education. Human potential for evil can be curbed by serious efforts to develop basic virtues like friendliness.

Friendliness means both being well disposed toward affectionate relationships with other persons and controlling hostile forces within oneself. Hostile instincts and drives are present to some degree in all human beings and make affectionate relationships with others difficult to sustain. If negative feelings are not taken into account and worked on, friendship doesn't have a chance. Persons who are full of resentment, for example, or are angry, and fail to recognize these feelings, cannot either establish friendships or maintain them. The same is true of persons dominated by envy. Certain attitudes push out the dispositions which lead to friendship.

If friendliness involves control of personal hostility, it requires understanding too, as one of its positive essential components. Being disposed to affection requires that I am able to look behind another person's acts, words, and behaviors, to the interior world of thoughts and feelings which lies behind them. But why? Simply to understand so as to be able to better control the other? No, just the opposite. Understanding makes it possible to judge others correctly. Seeing behind external acts to interior motives and feelings means, first of all, recognizing real interior dispositions and then situating the person's behavior in a broader context: one which involves the person's past childhood experiences, disappointments, tragedies, etc. Understanding grasps why a person acts one way or another, as well as the real meaning of the other's behavior. Such understanding is the only way to avoid reacting to the behavior of others strictly in kind. Tit for tat is the opposite of friendliness.

Understanding builds bridges between persons, whereas misunderstanding alienates and disposes for hurting. Sympathy and warm feelings flow from understanding, which remembers and learns from mistakes. But without understanding, a person is left with only a first impression, shot through with inadequate and downright mistaken interpretations. The alternative to understanding is lumping great varieties of people into those broad, black and white categories which typify prejudice. Prejudice, for example, is a form of misunderstanding.

Closely associated with understanding and the control of hostile forces is attentiveness to small details about the oftentimes cramped conditions in which we live. Because we bump into one another and cross one another's spheres of action, the potential for friction and anger is everywhere. One way to lessen this negative potential is by attending to the small needs of others. Small details of behavior, although they do not qualify as friendliness, certainly cut down on the enmity to which friendliness is opposed. Friendship is one of the great virtues or basic components for the good life, but not everything about good life has to do with greatness. Little things are very important. In the rush of medical practice, it is easy to let small courtesies slip. The doctor who works at being ethical has to keep a close eye on habits that undermine affection.

Friendliness also requires strength and a capacity for forgiveness. Life is full of disappointments caused more by persons than by events. Friendliness is frequently taken advantage of. People sometimes "use" their friends. If we live long enough we will be disappointed by a friend's behavior. Since this virtue, like all the rest, involves a certain consistency of behavior, the friendly person must be strong enough to continue making the effort to reach out even after disappointment. It is not enough to be well disposed once in a while. Friendliness requires the strength to forgive often. Understanding the complex psychological factors in patient hostility toward doctors should make it easier for the doctor to develop this strength.

Strength, yes, but friendliness cannot be too serious. The very idea of someone in total seriousness cultivating friendly attitudes is laughable. Talk of friendliness as control of hostility and strength suggests a serious side of the virtue, but the friendly person is not all serious. Friendliness disposes a person to positive affect toward others, but also to a sense of humor. Neither the self nor the other can be taken totally seriously. Friendliness has a lightness about it. It makes a person sensitive to the oddities in himself and others. The more pompous a person, the funnier he is because pomposity ignores the comic dimension of life. Friendliness disposes us to laugh, first at ourselves. The pompous doctor causes others to laugh, but doesn't have many friends.

One final remark about what friendliness means and how it is developed. There is an anticipatory quality to friendliness in the sense that the friendly person moves out toward the other. Friendliness makes friendship a pleasure and, consequently, disposes us to move with some ease toward establishing friendships. The limit of our human language and the complexities of the human world create imprecisions in our talk about an ethics of character and virtue. Characteristics like friendliness overlap with those of benevolence and respect. But the different virtues also speak to different features of a person's inner being. Friendliness is really different from respect and benevolence. It is warmer than benevolence and more active or initiating than respect.

Conclusion

Talk of virtues, character traits, moral education, and now friendliness sounds old fashioned, even to me. I sound almost as if I were writing religion instead of ethics. We don't talk about these topics anymore because religion is a dangerous topic in a secular society and because we have become busy with other concerns. This is more true of doctors than most others in our culture. Science and technology have focused attention on things rather than on persons. Doctors are focused on techniques and chemistry and mechanisms for the manipulation of nature. Concern about subjects has given way to concern about objects. For all these reasons, talk about virtue and character sounds old fashioned.

But not every development in science and technology has meant an improvement in life. One unhappy change which is easily seen in medicine and medical institutions is a hardening of the atmosphere. Human contact has become more coarse, and an older style of tenderness with patients has disappeared. Talk about medical ethics in the sense of the development of one's interior life through cultivation of virtues seems out of step. This approach "may be alright for romantic types," or "it would be nice if one had the time to think about such things." For the scientifically trained modern physician, concerns about the affective side of patient relations comes over as inessential, if not unreal. Real, for example, is what can be figured into the budget or produces immediate cash value. But is there any doubt that medical practice, which has become more coarse and less affective, has also become impoverished for both the doctor and the patient? When older doctors say that medicine is not fun anymore, they mean that it is no longer friendly and humane.

The contacts between doctor and patient have become objects of engineering science's time and motion studies, and every unproductive minute or movement is considered a loss. Only die-hard romantics deny the many improvements that have come from these engineering attitudes toward work. Only a blind positivist, however, would fail to see the losses which medicine has sustained along with the gains. The virtues of benevolence, honesty, respect and friendliness are all rooted in the needs of a person who is ill, and it is precisely these personal elements, that have suffered most from the changes which science and technology have wrought. At very least, it makes sense for the doctor to step back and take a look at the quality of his own life and the quality of the medicine he is practicing.

Even more than other ethical themes we have looked at, friendliness in medical practice seems to be an endangered virtue. Today's doctor/patient relationship leaves neither time nor the place for friendship. A doctor may respond "Oh, no, I am still very friendly and have authentically affectionate relations with my patients." This may be true, but if it is not, the doctor would be the last to know. To believe that all the cultural influences we just looked at have had no effect on medical behavior or on the quality of the doctor/patient relationship is foolish. No one can live within a culture that has become less personal and not be influenced. It may come as a shock to find out what ordinary patients think about their doctor's friendliness; not the special admiring patients, but the ordinary ones.

Notes

1. Paracelsus, *Spitalbuch,* I. Teil. (Translation mine).

2. Freud, Sigmund, *Studies on Hysteria.* (New York: Avon Books), 1966.

3. Seneca, *Moral Essays.* John W. Basore, trans., (Cambridge, MA: Harvard University Press), 1964.

6.

Access to Medical Help and the Virtue of Justice

It is easy to attend only to the surface of the doctor/patient relationship, and superficially this encounter appears to be a completely private affair. The doctor and the patient are private persons and meet in a private consulting room. They speak to one another privately, and away from witnesses. Private thoughts and feelings are shared by the patient, and the doctor is committed to guard the privacy of this communication. Patients choose a particular doctor for personal reasons, and in small town America they still pay their doctors' bills from private funds. Despite appearances, however, what takes place between the doctor and the patient is as social as it is ethical, affective, spiritual, or medical. Medical practice, in general, and the doctor/patient relationship in particular is indeed essentially social.

"Well," I can hear a reader say, "Really?" "And what is social about diabetes or cancer?" "What is social about the solitary person who happens to find himself ill?" "Doesn't every particular patient suffer an individualized form of an illness and suffer it alone, except for the help offered by the doctor?" Yes, but on the other hand, there is usually a genetic element in disease and genes are transmitted socially. In fact, genes form part of a gene pool, which is a social reality. In diagnosis, doctors take histories, not just to look for genetic factors, but to look for other social factors as well, which are implicated in "individual illnesses." Early childhood influences, family life, schooling, alimentation related to economic and ethnic background, all these are social factors.

At first view, cancer seems to be an individualized illness, but the more that is known about cancer, the more obvious its social features are. Certain types of cancer strike the rich, while others are more concentrated among the poor. Some national groups have higher incidences of certain cancer, while in others, the same cancers are unknown. What is true of cancer is true of other illnesses. Individuals get sick, but the roots of illness are in some form social and so are the ways in which illness is experienced. A person's social class, national origin, regional identification, profession, cultural or religious circle all have an influence on which illnesses are contracted and how illnesses are experienced.

The enormous popularity of books by anthropologists Ruth Benedict and Margaret Mead have created a fairly widespread awareness of the fact that different cultures have different ideas about illness. We know, for example, that in America, what is called an emotional illness in some African cultures may be considered a religious manifestation or even a badge of esteem. But even within our own culture, for every 1,000 biological or psychological disturbances, only 100 or so will be considered illness and sufficient reason for seeing a doctor. And the number of illness categories changes with time and is different in different groups. One interesting study done years ago on a college campus showed Jewish students and students majoring in economics called the doctor for upsets more often than any other group on campus.

If illness and patients have a social dimension, so do doctors. Are doctors today the same as they were 100 years ago? The idea of what it means to be a good doctor has changed. Medical education, too, has changed not just in scientific content, but in the moral formation given to doctors, and these changes are reflections of widespread changes that have taken place within our society.

It is obvious that doctors are not all the same. Some are aristocratic; others proletarian; most are middle class. These social differences affect the way a doctor practices medicine. Religious doctors (Protestant, Catholic, Jewish), secular or atheistic doctors, doctors working for the government or for a company, doctors involved in research groups: they all practice differently because of their association with different social groups. The fact that the doctor is educated at great social expense and exercises a considerable social power as a result of that education gives to every medical practitioner a distinct social dimension.

Social Aspects of the Doctor/Patient Relationship

If doctors and illnesses are socially conditioned, the doctor/patient relationship also has to be. A socially conditioned doctor and patient meet in a time and place at least partially determined by social factors. Doctor and patient each have social roles to perform and expectations to meet. For example, patients in American society are usually relieved of their normal social obligations for as long as they remain ill. The doctor is the person authorized by society to certify illness and officially to dispense the patient from these obligations. The patient's freedom from work obligations is based on the social assumption that patients are not responsible for their illness. The patient is, however, obliged to want to get better and to try to do so by going to the doctor and cooperating with the doctor's therapeutic interventions. Doctors are also obliged by society to undertake the work of curing and to make sure that patients do not derive anti-social advantage from their illness. In a society like the Soviet Union, as well as in many non-technological societies, the social system dictates different social expectations and different social roles for the doctor and patient.

Besides the roles and expectations dictated by society, the doctor/patient relationship is social in itself. Its structure is social. Medical diagnosis, for example, which seems a thoroughly private act, is carried out with resources which are different for patients in the military than for patients belonging to an HMO. Insurance companies will pay for some tests but not for others, and thereby influence the way a diagnosis is conducted. The DRGs are a socially approved set of diagnostic categories which, in these days, have everything to do with the way patients are treated. Even something like the popularity or loss of popularity of certain diagnostic procedures influence their use. At one time, X-rays were very popular and used very frequently. Social influence may not be the most evident or the strongest element in medical diagnosis, but certainly it is there.

If society influences diagnostic procedures, imagine what it does to therapy. Certain medicines and even certain surgical procedures come in and out of style. Some procedures are popular with some groups, but not with others. Societies in the sense of particular groups to which a patient may belong (HMO, military, Blue Cross/Blue Shield, Medicare, Medicaid) will have something to do with the type of treatment received. Even different hospitals are different social groups (research, university, private, for-profit) and they too, influence treatment procedures. But the major socially rooted difference in the way patients are treated derives from the patient's socioeconomic status. Not only is there a medicine for the rich and a medicine for the poor (somewhat comparable to the medicine for citizens and medicine for slaves in Ancient Greece), but there is treatment or no treatment, depending on socioeconomic factors (Estimates place the number of persons without health insurance and, therefore, without access to treatment, as high as 15 percent of the American population).

Decisions which patients make about treatment are obviously influenced by social forces. Family, for example, often have a considerable influence on patient decisions. Sometimes without reason, doctors look to family for decisions which the patient has every right to make. More remotely, church groups, ethnic background and socioeconomic status have considerable influence on the way patients choose and even the way disease and treatment information is communicated to patients. Doctors talk differently to patients from different social groups and classes. Finally, the affective dimension of the doctor/patient encounter, more than anything else, is influenced by the fact that hundreds of technicians now deliver medical treatment. The old friendship between the doctor and the patient has all but disappeared in many social contexts.

Today, the essentially social doctor/patient relationship is undergoing an even more intense socialization. Patients, who since the earliest times have thought of medical care as a benefit, now consider it a right and one automatically enjoyed by everyone. The very appearance of illness, instead of being considered a misfortune becomes for some, a violation of a "right to health" for which compensation is owed. This new "right" extends to organic infirmities of the gravest sort, and also to minor functional problems. The books of Thomas Szasz, which ignore the inherent distortions of psychiatric illnesses in order to convert them into purely social labels, reflect an increased socialization of medicine in our time.[1]

Forms of Increased Socialization

Movement away from the private in medicine is most obvious when the forms of practice are looked at. More and more frequently, medical practice is some form of group practice. The old private practitioner is now more likely to be a member of a team. If a doctor practices in a hospital, this team will have members from outside the medical profession: social workers, psychologists, and even perhaps a medical ethicist. The truly private practioner is an endangered species.

Private practitioners used to send their patients to privately owned drug stores. Now the drug store itself reflects an increased socialization of medicine. Medications that only a few years ago were prepared by a pharmacist upon presentation of a doctor's prescription can now be found on row after row of shelves. People treat themselves today with powerful over-the-counter hypnotics, analgesics, tranquilizers, laxatives, medicines for heart, blood pressure, colds, allergies, etc., and this extensive socialization of therapy has already begun to be seen in diagnosis. Many diagnostic kits are on the market, and many others will follow. The diagnostic technologies which now feed back numbers and require translation by some techician to more meaningful lay language can be made to speak directly to the patient. Therapy, socialized to the point of not requiring a physician, may be followed by diagnosis socialized in the same way.

But the clearest example of this trend toward increased socialization is the hospital itself. Stanley Reiser, in his book on contemporary medical practice[2] counted over two hundred medical technicians operating in modern medical centers. American hospitals which started out providing nursing care gradually added one new service after another. Pharmacies, autopsy facilities, pathology labs, chemistry labs, microbiology labs, radiology facilities, etc., have generated an army of medical technicians, all of whom are involved in patient care. It is even hard to think of a type of social service that one does not find in today's hospitals. The hospital itself has become a society, a city within a city, and the subject matter of countless sociological studies.

The conclusion from this quick survey of medical practice today is unavoidable. The old model of medicine, as a solitary meeting of doctor and patient as if on a deserted island, is every day less realistic. Illnesses are social, physicians are social, therapy and diagnosis are social, hospitals are social institutions, and therefore the doctor/patient relationship is social.

Socialization of Medical Care Delivery

The one aspect of this widespread reality on which I want to focus, has to do with the delivery of medical care. We have already mentioned that in ancient Greece, a different type of medical care was provided for citizens and slaves. In modern America, certain diagnostic and therapeutic modalities are accessible only to the economically well situated. And the differences in medical care accessibility seem to be widening rather than narrowing. An already substantial number of persons in America, the medically disinherited, do not even get a poor man's care; they get no care at all. This change is one that normally developed moral consciences find difficult to accept as they find it difficult to accept that poor people are used as experimental subjects for high priced procedures which later will be available only for the rich (for example, artificial hearts). But what can be done about it? Frankly, I don't know. My limited goal is to call attention to the fact that in order to be a good doctor, the physician today must at least recognize the strong social character of the doctor/patient relationship and then give some attention to the virtue of justice which will dispose him or her to try to do something to address the social problems of medicine.

Doctors alone cannot solve the enormous social problem of care for the poor in our society, but no solution will ever be found which does not include physicians. Doctors are not the bad guys who created the problem, but certainly they will be the prime targets of a moral rebellion which can be expected if the problem is left unattended. Many of the attitudinal changes in patients already mentioned can be understood as instances of a patient rebellion already underway. Medical associations have paid more attention to fighting the socialization of medicine than to understanding the complex involvements of medicine in modern society. The socialization process is real and in some sense responds to a bottom line demand in this and every advanced society that sick people get adequate medical treatment. If basic delivery breaks down, there will be a widespread social upheaval, beginning with rebellion against the system of medical delivery which leaves large segments of the population with inadequate to non-existent medical care. This problem cannot continue to be left in the hands of experts. A more extensive involvement is required.

When people are seriously ill so as to put them in danger of death, and they know that medical treatments for their problem are available, they are not going to accept sickness and death with resignation. The wonders of modern medicine are too well publicized to go unnoticed, and people who are suffering naturally want what they know will help them. The rebellion of the masses who found themselves outside established levels of medical care over the last one hundred years has produced radical changes in the medical delivery system of all the advanced technological nations. Generally, these changes have been in the direction of socialization, with some basic level of medical care guaranteed for each citizen. This level is different in different countries and what, in most of the existing systems is considered "adequate," would be seen as shockingly inadequate by most Americans. But even in America, pressure is being generated to define a level of adequate care to which every citizen has a right. Once this is done, some adjustment in the American system of delivery will have to be made, and doctors will have everything to do with whether an adjustment toward the poor and toward primary care actually works out in practice.

The Soviet system of total state control not only provides inferior medical care, but simply would not fit with the American experience. Besides, it is in such chaos that it has fallen below even Soviet expectations. And the once highly touted intermediary socialization systems in places like England and Scandinavia are now showing serious problems and major deficiencies. It nevertheless remains true that too many people in America find themselves either outside or on the fringes of this otherwise impressive medical system. We cannot forget that half of the persons called up for military service during the Second World War were rejected for medical reasons and two-thirds of those rejected had problems which could have been prevented with adequate medical attention. Any social system for delivering medical care will require the attention of those people who care most about helping the sick: the doctors. And what disposes the doctor to give his attention to this problem is the virtue of justice. A thirst for justice developed in the doctor will not, by itself, solve the delivery problem, but this problem will not be solved without it.

No matter how economically generous and efficiently organized the medical delivery system for poor people, it will not work without personal commitments from doctors to the justice issue. The subjective moral formation of the good doctor is as important as the developed sense of civil morality in the general population. People have to care about justice before good solutions will be found. Doctors have to be just for any just system of health delivery to work.

Improving the Present System

Perhaps the place for doctors to start caring about justice is precisely where they presently find themselves. A new national health policy is not the only way to bring about a more just system. Even in the best medical facilities as presently organized (the clinics, small hospitals, group and private practices), substantial improvements are needed in the way medical care is delivered. The worst aspect of totally socialized delivery systems is the ugly bureaucratization which turns even those patients who gain most from them into humiliated paupers. But something similar can occur in our private medical institutions. Nothing can match the dehumanization of patients in large, overcrowded facilities in the Soviet Union or other Soviet bloc states, but patients can also be dehumanized here. Receptionists, nurses and secretaries can create a system which turns patients into numbers and forms, and then makes them wait for hours to see the doctor. The few short, hurried minutes with the doctor further diminish the patient, because the assembly line treatment ignores both the patient's anxiety and the importance he or she gives to the illness. Simply put, something is wrong with our system. No wonder so many patients are disappointed after a visit to the doctor.

But isn't this just picky and petty complaining? Does it merit being included in a chapter about justice and health care delivery? Is waiting such a big deal? No one will disagree that waiting joined to an all too short visit with the doctor are characteristic of our delivery system. We wait to talk to the receptionist, wait to see the nurse, wait to see the doctor, wait to get the results of tests, and always feel that the wait was unfair when it is compared to the time we are attended by the doctor. The doctor's time is valuable, no doubt about it. But is the time of every patient valueless? If patients in socialized systems and clients in welfare systems are dehumanized by being made to wait in long lines for a short visit with state bureaucrats, then something similar happens to patients even in the best outlets of the American delivery system. The treatment of patients in large, high-tech medical centers which serve as teaching hospitals for medical schools, is far worse from a human standpoint than what goes on in the small clinic. What happens in both types of delivery outlets is far removed from what it means to treat the patient as a person.

A Virtue of Justice

No virtue is easily acquired, but special efforts will be needed for the physician to acquire the virtue of justice, because traditionally very little attention has been paid to justice in medical training. Naturally, it is difficult to develop a character trait corresponding to a dimension of the medical act that has largely been ignored. Traditionally, doctors have paid attention to what they considered important; i.e., real science rather than the issues of a so-called social science. As a profession, medicine is deeply involved in society and, indeed, in politics. But professionally, doctors have adopted an attitude toward both which is reminiscent of the American Puritans, who considered one and the other slightly sinful. Like the early Puritans, modern doctors can afford to ignore social issues because, as a matter of fact, through the lobbying efforts of medical association leaders, they exercise considerable social power.

The power of doctors, like that of other professionals in our society, comes from the important specialized knowledge they have. In monarchical societies, power depended upon blood, but in contemporary technological cultures, knowledge is what counts. The old aristocrats simply inherited their power and with it a strong sense of responsibility for the society in which their power was exercised. Present-day professional power holders, however (doctors among them), have little sense of social responsibility. Consequently, professional power is exercised almost exclusively for personal gain and this despite the fact that doctors' powerful knowledge was acquired either at public expense or at least with considerable public support. Developing a sense of social responsibility will not be easy, but neither should doctors be considered "lost causes" as critics have claimed.

The first difficulty to be overcome has to do with understanding what justice means. When we speak of friendliness or honesty or even respectfulness, most people have an immediate commonsense understanding of what these words mean. The word "justice," however, may likely bring to mind something that lawyers are involved with, but not doctors, and not ordinary people in their day-to-day life. The term "justice," like its cognate "just," seems quite removed from personal characteristics and from acquired habits. Honesty is immediately recognized as a personally appropriated good way of being, but not justice. And yet, even a very small child who has little or no experience with honesty has a strongly developed sense of what is just. Paradoxically, justice and just are both the most abstract and the most concrete of all the moral categories.

All of us have experienced something comparable to the following scene. Children are sitting around the table celebrating a birthday in the family, and it comes time to divide the cake. The mother cuts a piece, and as it is passed along from child to child, it is carefully examined by each. Even before the distribution is complete, one of the children complains because "he got a bigger piece than I did." If the mother tries to "even things out," what was up until that point a nice party can quickly turn into a family war. The child who originally may or may not have received a bigger piece will, himself, begin to complain if any attempt is made to change the original distribution. Every child at the table not only has an unshakable sense that the only right thing is a perfectly even distribution of the cake, but anything less will be experienced as painfully wrong. "It's not fair" will be the cry, followed perhaps by a decision not to eat any cake at all rather than to be satisfied with something less than what others received.

Or after dinner, the father settles into his favorite chair to read the paper and reaches for his pipe. The child who recognizes that habitual move immediately asks if she can light the pipe. The father agrees. Just as quickly, another child protests, "You let her light the pipe instead of me. It isn't fair."

Justice, in its most primitive form, is understood as fairness, and each child has an unshakable sense that the only right thing is rigorously fair treatment. A classical philosophical definition of justice as "giving to everyone his due" is not far removed from that very early moral experience. We are concerned here with justice in the sense of fair distribution of medical goods and services. The problem which presses most insistently upon the social conscience of the medical profession is not simply that some get more or better medical treatment than others, but that some get the very best treatment available in the world and others get none at all. The inequalities that exist do not work to the benefit of the least advantaged.[3]

The Components of Justice

Corresponding to the objective morality of fair distribution is the virtue of justice in the sense of the personal appropriation of justice and fairness. The virtue of justice refers to that strength of character which is required to do what is fair to other persons. The virtue of justice, like a standard of justice, is something real: a subjective, but real disposition which carries over into habitual objective acts of giving to others what is their due.

Jesus may have said it better than anyone else, when he referred to the virtue of justice in terms of an urge: Blessed are they that hunger and thirst after justice (Matt 5:6). This moral virtue is compared physically to hunger and thirst; both strong and very elementary urgings. Besides fair and just acts, there are urges, leanings, dispositions which have to be cultivated and made part of a person's character. These subjective forces make it possible to keep trying over and over again to make the treatment of other individuals fair. What is theoretically considered to be due the other person will change as will the historical understanding of fairness and justice, but the root of the virtue of justice remains this primitive urge for fairness.

The virtue of justice is something as real as the objectively just acts in which it terminates. It is the appropriation of fairness into one's own character, a refinement of a natural urge to treat others fairly. This refinement is carried out by free and intelligent choices. It is one thing to cultivate the urge for fairness; another to know what fairness is. All virtue involves the use of prudence and intelligence because virtues are refinements of human persons who cannot help but be in the world in an intelligent way. There is no such thing as blind virtue or ignorant virtue or unconscious virtue. Some people are more naturally inclined than others to the practice of certain good acts, but to qualify as virtue, a personality trait must involve the use of intelligence and be the product of free choice. What is true of virtue in general is even more true of justice. The virtue of justice is penetrated and tempered by intelligence.

Intelligence is an integral part of the virtue of justice because fairness in the sense of adjusting available good so that everyone receives "what is his due" is a painfully difficult task. What is due the other? What is the other's share? What does the other have a right to? Due, share, right are always changing with the historical circumstances and with the theories which gain acceptability in a culture. Intelligence that is legally, economically, and humanly sophisticated is required even to approach this complex issue. In a field as complex as medical care, a specialized intelligence is especially required as a prelude to the virtue of justice which disposes us not to thoughts or concepts, but to acts of fairness. As far as doctors are concerned, the virtue of justice disposes to concrete acts of giving what is due to patients, and obviously such a disposition requires a cultivated intelligence.

The Object of Justice

What is a person's due or right when it comes to medical care? Certainly, it is not just what one is able to pay for from private funds. Such an idea of due and right would leave a society radically split between a few who could get the best care and the rest who could afford either inadequate or no care at all. Such a system would be too unequal, and justice has something to do with equality as we saw in the examples of the children. To be equal, things have to be weighed and balanced. The root word for weighing is *pensare* or *pesare,* which we find in English words like com*pensa*tion and recom*pense*: words which are closely linked with equality and justice. Since justice and equality even things up when they are out of balance, the virtue of justice disposes us to do just that. The doctor today, with a developed sense of justice as part of his personality, has to be concerned and working to even up, or to rebalance an unequal system, and to compensate or recompense those who have less.

This balancing and evening up, to which the virtue of justice disposes us, has to be done over and over again. Justice is not satisfied by one act of equalizing. It must carry over into repeated acts of balancing, compensating, and giving what is due to people who have little or nothing. Compensation and recompensation are part of justice because the right balance never has been established and never will be. The distribution of goods is always out of balance to some degree, which is why the virtue of justice disposes to repeated acts aimed at fairness. At one time or another, we are all either debtors or creditors. What the Marxist system says about the establishment of justice at the end of socialism is simply not true. Human beings will never arrive at a state of social order when balancing and equaling will no longer be required. What Jesus said is not only true to the facts, but remains good advice to the physician: thirst after justice, try to make things more fair in medicine, work to overcome the more blatant forms of inequality and maldistribution of medical services. Precisely because objective justice is never achieved, the virtue of justice struggles and hungers for better balance.

Why be Just?

But why make this effort? Why not simply look out for oneself and forget about this problem of fairness to others? Let others take care of themselves! With all the modern day doctor is faced with, does it make any sense to try to become conversant with the complexities of medical distribution, in order to work for a more just and balanced system? The answer is yes, and for many different reasons. From a purely selfish perspective, the alternative to doctors with more developed moral dispositions toward justice is a gradual worsening of the present imbalance in distribution and a sharpening of the antagonisms against the medical profession. Patient rebellion has already forced changes and will force still more. Many of the possible changes on the horizon will worsen both medical practice and the situation of the doctor, and so it makes sense to get out in front on this issue. Instead of being the "bad guy," resisting every proposal for meeting the needs of the least advantaged, the medical profession can come up with plans reflective of a more widespread thirst and hunger for justice among doctors. Until now, the proposals coming from the medical associations have not created the impression of professionals anxious to create a better system for the least advantaged. It may not be true, but they appear to a lay public as more protective of doctors than of patients.

Another reason is more philosophical. Human beings need a certain number of material and spiritual goods to become fully themselves. Beside the material goods required for physical survival, people need the many basic goods referred to in the nineteenth century declarations of human rights, the so-called second generation social rights. Without basic goods, human beings lose their humanity: they can maintain neither their dignity nor their human stature. Say what we will, more than negative freedoms or first generation formal rights (e.g., to be left alone, privacy) are needed to live a decent life. Medical care is one such critical good, especially in technological societies where most people have to work in order to live. If any Americans today lack adequate medical care, they suffer dehumanization.

What is adequate care? The content of this term needs to be worked out by experts who know what monies this culture can make available and what limits will be required on specialized procedures to make the monies available for basic services. Every American does not need access to artificial hearts, but does need to be treated for broken legs, apendicitis, hemorrhages, ulcers and the like. Adequate care is required for sick people to be human, and the system which provides it requires the doctors, themselves, to be human. A badly imbalanced medical delivery system dehumanizes both the patients and the doctors.

Because the problem of fair distribution and adequate treatment is so overwhelming, an individual doctor may be tempted to do nothing about it. And yet the efforts of individual doctors help when, out of a more developed sense of justice, they do things for poor patients. The virtue of justice, like its sister virtue charity, begins at home. Doctors can be more just in their offices, in their hospitals, with their work for social services of their community. Even without another degree in medical economics, an individual practitioner can recognize certain situations close to home which violate a sense of fairness and do something to remedy them. Every doctor can begin by looking at the way people are treated in his or her own office.

The virtue of justice, which derives from the inherently social dimension of the doctor/patient relationship, has its ultimate roots in the very nature of human persons. Theories of moral development show how this primitive moral urge for justice changes and evolves toward a thirst for and a work toward a fairer social system. Because the virtue of justice is so basic to human beings, for doctors to leave this personality dimension underdeveloped is to condemn themselves to an unattractive form of ethical retardation. Good doctors are both more attractive human beings and better professionals. A deep-seated commitment to justice will, in addition, bring the doctor into contact with the limits of all human efforts to do the good and raise religious questions suggested by those limits. It is to these questions that we now turn.

Notes

1. Szasz, Thomas. *Psychiatric Justice*, (New York: Macmillan), 1965. See also, Thomas Szasz, *The Ethics of Psychoanalysis: The Theory and Method of Autonomous Psychotherapy*, (New York: Basic Books), 1965; and Thomas Szasz, *Law, Liberty, and Psychiatry: An Inquiry into the Social Uses of Mental Health Practices*, (New York: Macmillan), 1963.

2. Reiser, Stanley. *Medicine and the Reign of Technology*, (Cambridge University Press), 1978; and Stanley Reiser, *The Machine at the Bedside: Strategies for using Technology in Patient Care*, (New York: Cambridge University Press), 1984.

3. This is one of the basic principles of an important formalistic, Kantian style theory of justice, developed by John Rawls, a Harvard philosopher. Rawls, John., *A Theory of Justice*, (Cambridge, Mass.: Harvard University Press), 1971. An opposing view of justice which is most concerned with maximizing freedom, and less with the plight of poor people, is articulated by another Harvard philosopher, Robert Nozich. Nozich, Robert., *Anarchy, State, Utopia*, (New York: Basic Books), 1974. An application of Nozich's view to the world of medicine is articulated by H. Tristram Englehardt. Englehardt, Tristram H., *The Foundations of BioEthics*, (New York: Oxford University Press), 1986.

7.

Doctors as Priests, and the Virtue of Religion

As strange as it may seem to us today to link religion with medicine, or priesthood with doctoring, historically, the two have always been closely connected. In primitive societies, we find one person who functioned as tribal chief, priest and physician. Joining the doctor's role in history with those of leader and priest gave a prestige to medicine which continues to our day. Jokes about doctors mistaking themselves for kings or gods may actually go back a very long way.

The early and enduring association of medicine with religion and priesthood gave an other-worldly quality to medical knowledge— presumably it came from the gods. Rules which doctors laid down for patients also took on characteristics similar to religious norms. Even in primitive societies, there were different kinds of workers, but those who treated the ill and wrestled with death were not like the rest of men. Doctors, historically, were distinguished by three characteristics: 1) Because they were chosen from the community, they enjoyed a higher status or privilege. 2) Associated with specialness and separateness, they enjoyed civil and criminal impunity. 3) Naturally, they enjoyed and exercised authority.[1] Privilege, impunity, and authority have endured as characteristics of the doctor throughout history. A tendency in our society to sue the doctor has created serious social problems, but to doctors this development is an unprecedented affront and their reactions are expressed in terms of sacrilege and tones of blasphemy. The religious quality of the doctors' reaction to the malpractice craze may be better understood by remembering some medical history.

Hebrew Cultures

Western people are most familiar with the ancient culture of Israel, and there we can see examples of what occurred in many other primitive societies. Moses was the political leader of Israel, the priestly mediator between God and man, and finally, the one people looked to for help in times of sickness. Moses ruled the people, communed with God and cured the sick. Later on, a separate tribe was designated to carry out priestly functions, but the link between priesthood and medicine remained. The Israelite priests imposed rules of life on the people in the name of God himself, and among them were medical rules. Priests decreed both what was right and wrong,[2] and what was pure and impure. They applied religious sanctions to dietary regulations. And they diagnosed those who were ill and distinguished the ill from the healthy.[3]

Interestingly enough, the physician/priest relationship was carried over both into the standards of priesthood and the rules governing the selection of priests. To be a priest one had to be healthy, especially in the sense of being without what then were called "defects in the bloodline." Sanctity of the priesthood was one theme of the *Book of Leviticus*, and, in chapter 21, we find a list of medical defects that disqualify a person otherwise destined to be a priest. We are used to hearing about aristocratic blue blood which was required to rule, but there was also a priestly blood (purple?), and it had to be healthy.

> The Lord said to Moses, speak to Aaron and tell him; none of your descendents of whatever generation who has any defects shall come forward to offer up the food of his God. Therefore, he who has any of the following defects many not come forward: he who is blind, or lame, or who has any disfigurement or malformation, or a crippled foot or hand, or who is humpbacked, or weakly, or walleyed, or who is afflicted with eczema, ringworm or hernia. No descendant of Aaron, the priest, who has any such defect may draw near to offer up the oblation of the Lord; on account of his defect, he may not draw near to offer up the food of his God.[4]

It would be wrong to suggest that only priests were doctors. Alongside the priestly doctors who enjoyed privilege, impunity and authority, there were "lower class" physicians with a social position similar to that of carpenters or blacksmiths. These "secular" doctors enjoyed none of the privileges of the priestly group. Modern physicians may actually be the historical successors of lower class doctors, surgeons, and pharmacists, but the social characteristics of today's doctors are more in the tradition of their priestly predecessors.

The Greeks

About one thousand years later, (depending upon the periodization of Moses and the first Hippocratic doctors), a non-priestly group of physicians moved from the lower social ranks of craftsmen to positions near the top of the Greek social ladder. The Hippocratic physicians were secular and scientific, but they gained a social position close to philosophers who were the "priests" of Greece's classical period. Hippocratic writings can neither be intelligently interpreted nor adequately understood without keeping in mind their "priestly" characteristics.

Enormous value was placed upon the human body in Greek civilization, and one reason for the ever higher social status of Hippocratic doctors was their involvement with the body. Hippocratic doctors adopted a technical approach to body, illness and health, and "technical" for the Greeks meant systematic and methodological. These doctors were different from other healers in that they knew both what to do and why it needed to be done. Their "scientific" approach provided credibility for what these doctors did, and led medicine to become one of the culture's basic institutions. What philosophy did for the mind, Hippocratic medicine did for the body, and this association with philosophy in the sense of "knowing why" or understanding gave it real prestige. It seems strange to us that these secular-scientific Hippocratic doctors would understand themselves and their work in priestly terms, but the fact that they did so can hardly be disputed.

A priestly tone literally leaps out of the Hippocratic Oath which has served as an ideal statement of medical behavior for almost 2,500 years. In the Oath, medicine is portrayed as a difficult art, the practice of which is inseparable from priestly moral standards:

"I will use treatment to help the sick."

"I will neither do harm nor commit injustice."

"I will keep both my life and my art pure and holy."

"In whatever house I enter, I will enter to help the sick and I will abstain from intentional wrong-doing and harm, especially from sexual acts with either men or women, slaves or free."

"Whatever I might see or hear in the course of treatment, or even outside, if it should not be divulged, I will keep silence, holding such things to be holy secrets."[5]

Being committed to the good of others, to a rigid and high standard of social conduct, to avoiding harm and injustice, are priestly virtues. And besides, physicians make a specific promise of holiness, both in life and in work. In addition, there is the "priestly secret," the promise to treat as "confessional" material, even things learned inside and outside medical practice. Whether or not the code's priestly flavor derives from an association of Hippocratic doctors with the Pythagorean religious sect has not been proven. What is clear, however, is the fact that the ancient predecessors of today's scientific/technical doctors definitely thought of themselves in priestly terms.

This can be seen in many other texts throughout the Hippocratic corpus. *The Law* is an important little document which talks about the education of a good physician. It ends with these words: "Things, however, that are holy are revealed only to men who are holy. The profane may not learn them until they have been initiated into the mysteries of science."[6] Here we have an explicit reference to the dual identities of priest-scientist. Hippocratic physicians who set themselves apart from the temple doctors by their technical/scientific approach maintained a sense of their sacredness.

In practicing medicine, the Hippocratic doctor comes into contact with, and actually encounters, the sacred. The divine, the ethical and the rational were considered to be the essential characteristics of *nature* (*physis*). The body, in fact, was thought of as nature itself in miniature (*microcosmos*). The doctor then handled the sacred, much like the priest, and an awareness of this is expressed throughout the Hippocratic writings.

In the first chapter of another Hippocratic work, *The Physician*, we find an outline of qualities and virtues required of the physician:

> The dignity of a physician requires that he should look healthy, and as plump as nature intended him to be; for the common crowd consider those who are not of this excellent bodily condition to be unable to take care of others. Then he must be clean in person, well dressed, and anointed with sweet-smelling unguents that are not in any way suspicious. This, in fact, is pleasing to patients. The prudent man must also be careful of certain moral considerations—not only to be silent, but also of a great regularity of life, since thereby his reputation will be greatly enhanced; he must be a gentleman in character, and being this he must be grave and kind to all. For an

over-forward obtrusiveness is despised, even though it may be very useful. Let him look to the liberty of action that is his; for when the same things are rarely presented to the same persons there is content [Translation not clear]. In appearance, let him be of a serious but not harsh countenance; for harshness is taken to mean arrogance and unkindness, while a man of uncontrolled laughter and excessive gaiety is considered vulgar, and vulgarity especially must be avoided. In every social relation he will be fair, for fairness must be of great service. The intimacy also between physician and patient is close. Patients, in fact, put themselves into the hands of their physician, and at every moment he meets women, maidens and possessions very precious indeed. So towards all these self-control must be used. Such then should the physician be, both in body and in soul.[7]

To be silent, ordered, of good character, serious, just, etc., these are high moral requirements. The Hippocratic physicians imposed upon themselves not just priestly commitments, priestly standards of unselfishness and priestly secrecy, but many other character traits which gave physicians a priestly ethos and held them to moral standards higher than persons involved in secular trades and professions. The early medical ethics was an ethics of high priestly character. The doctor had both to be good and to appear upright in the community.[8]

Christian Civilization

The philosophies of Plato and Aristotle were not the only Greek accomplishments that found easy access into Christian civilization. In the Hippocratic Oath, pagan religious references were replaced by Christian ones, but neither the tone nor the substance of the oath was changed as it became the standard ethical code for physicians throughout Christian civilization. In fact, St. Jerome, in outlining the duties of Christian priests, referred to visitation of the sick and reminded priests of the Hippocratic Oath and the obligation of priestly secrecy. The priestly virtues of Hippocratic doctoring were even used as models for how Christian priests should behave. Christian doctors retained strong similarities to priests long after their professionalization during the Middle Ages.

With the requirement of a university education and approval by an examining tribunal, medicine became a lay profession.[9] But the medieval university was an ecclesiastical institution, organized along the lines of a pre-Vatican II Catholic seminary. There were only five faculties in the university and three of the five (philosophy, theology, and canon law) were for training priests. Civil law and medicine were for laymen, but students in both received an education similar to candidates for the priesthood, especially where ethics and character formation were concerned. Doctors and judges were held to the same moral standards as priests. Judges today continue to reflect in dress and demeanor their historical priestly associations. Doctors do, too, but with white rather than black robes and with different ritualistic requirements for proper meetings.

The history of medicine and especially of medical ethics can be understood as an attempt on the part of a profession to go in opposite directions at the same time. Medicine took a giant step in the direction of becoming an independent lay profession when Henry VIII established the Royal College of Physicians in London which was free of either state or church control. There, doctors took control of their own education and standards for entrance into the profession. At the same time, sixteenth century English physicians distanced themselves from other "professional" groups which had formed to advance their own economic interests. Doctors, in fact, were like others who performed services for money. Unlike lawyers and merchants, however, they retained their priestly commitments to the good of society and their patients, and they kept their sense of themselves as belonging to a monopolistic priestly caste.[10]

When Adam Smith and liberal economists attacked the medical monopoly for violating the dogmas of free trade, doctors counter-attacked by insisting that medicine was not a business. Where human life and health are the issues, doctors argued, what is required is priestly commitment to the good of others, and priestly virtues on the part of practitioners. Without such priestliness, sick people would be vulnerable to exploitation by quacks. Then (and now), an ideology of priesthood and priestly standards of virtue were used as justification for treating physicians differently. Doctors won that argument.

But there were two sides of medical practice, and that bipolarity has not disappeared: ethical standards straight out of the priestly tradition, and a practice which involved the provision of services for monetary gain. The traditional codes of medical ethics reflect this dual orientation. Libertarian ethicists attack medical codes as self-serving and patronizing. But the high-sounding moral qualities, to which physicians oblige themselves in the codes, have to be understood before being criticized as out of harmony with contemporary standards. The codes were, and continue to be, reflections of a priestly tradition which shows that physicians have always been held to ethical standards higher than other professionals.

The ambiguity embedded in the priestly tradition of medicine is a real one. And so is the tension between priestly privileges and the social forces which resent the doctor's privilege, impunity and authority. Well into the nineteenth century doctors, like priests, were exempt from paying taxes, and justifications for such a privilege always took the form of an ideology of priesthood. "Doctors, like priests, are arbiters of death;" "They hold the very destiny of a person in their hands;" "Doctors are not held to explain their actions before human tribunals;" "Only God and their conscience is their judge." These were claims made historically by physicians in defense of their privileged place in society.[11] Any suggestion of putting limits on the doctor's immunity from court testimony, for example, brought an immediate reference to the priestly character of physician obligation to secrecy and to the profession's ruination if any changes were permitted. Doctors in the nineteenth century were said not to earn pay for their work, but rather, like priests, they were given a "stipend" or an "honorarium." And only the doctor could set the amount because only he "knew the time and effort which went into treatment." It was even argued that doctors were more priestly than priests, because "they cured body and soul;" "they risked their lives and often lost their lives" in order to do good for others.

The Modern Doctor: More Priestly Than Ever

"Well," the reader will be thinking, "those days are gone." Maybe doctors were once trained like priests, held to the same moral standards as priests, and enjoyed the same privilege, impunity and authority as priests, but all that ended in the twentieth century. Certainly legal impunity is gone. And so is the older system of retribution. Most doctors outside the United States, in fact, work for a government. Even in America, the free-standing, independent medical practitioner has become an endangered species. Finally, most modern doctors are specialists. They receive their patients from others, and send the patients back after problems associated with their organ specialty have been reviewed. Specialists certainly don't have a chance to be very priestly, and even family doctors have given up priestly pretense.

However, I think the opposite can be convincingly argued. Despite movement away from medieval priestly identifications toward secularity, doctors today are more priestly than ever. One could say that doctors are the only priests of our secular society. And here I do not refer to the obviously priestly role of today's psychiatrist, psychoanalyst, and the legions of spin-off therapists who practice a secularized, spiritual direction.

Medical doctors today are the priests of our secular society because health has taken the place of salvation, and the doctor is the only mediator of this new essential value. And doctors today exercise real priestly authority in the sense of laying down the rules of life: dictating what life is and how it should be lived. In religious societies, priests laid down the law for every aspect of life. Then, with the secularization process, judges, presidents, and prime ministers imposed a civil rather than a divine law. But in the twentieth century, neither traditional priests nor legislators have the authority of doctors. Once physical well-being becomes the goal of life, doctors are not like priests; they become priests. Not unlike priests in religious societies down through the years, modern doctors lay down rules of life for everyone.

Is there any doubt that physical well-being is the modern secular substitute for religion and salvation? When I studied theology in the 1940s and 1950s, the moral textbooks were preoccupied with the issue of religious scrupulosity. Catholic priests, especially, were given extensive theoretical and practical training in recognizing and treating the scrupulous person because religious scrupulosity was a big problem. But when, dear reader, was the last time you heard of a religiously scrupulous person? Obsessiveness has not disappeared. There are as many obsessives now as there ever were. But the vast majority are obsessed about the new understanding of salvation: health and physical well-being. The scrupulous penitent has given way to the health nut. Now it is the doctor/priest who has to handle "scrupulosity."

Only doctors successfully wrapped themselves in the mantle of modern science and, as a result, acquired impressive priestly powers at the expense of other traditional professions like law and priesthood. Now it's the doctor who lays down the norms for life and not just in the area of bodily health. Whatever the doctor says goes, outside as well as inside the hospital. Medical professionals direct the way we eat, exercise, work, sleep, raise children, educate the young and establish moral standards. The popular morning news programs feature doctors who tell us the latest findings about physical and emotional well-being. Handsome doctors tell us about medicine and also about how to handle stress, early childhood, adolescence, marriage, sex, Christmas depression, conflicts at work, moral conflict, and any crisis we face nationally or internationally. They exude priestly advice.

I recently saw a front page headline in our local paper, *Erie Daily Times,* which read, "Study Calls for Aggressive Use of Sex Education." This Associated Press story concerned a study of teenage pregnancy. A doctor, Daniel D. Federman of Harvard Medical School, chaired the study and concluded that "the major strategy for reducing unintended pregnancy must be the encouragement of diligent contraceptive use by all sexually active teenagers." Dr. Federman said that existing programs were ineffective and that making contraceptives available to teenagers did not encourage early sex. Obviously, this doctor's report was prescribing an ethics and not a medicine. It was laying down priestly norms for the life of individuals and for society and will have a major social impact on school districts all around the nation. The next morning, a doctor on the *Today Show* was showing fathers how to care for small children, and he laid down rules for being a loving parent. Hardly a day passes when doctors do not use their priestly authority on American people.

Medicine in modern American life does far more than cure disease. The M.D. degree is more authoritative than a Ph.D., and if a person had a clear cut plan for making social changes in American life, he or she would be well advised to study medicine. Even if there were no intention of practicing, the M.D. degree would make it possible to speak with authority in America, as traditional priests did in another time.

Religion in the Doctor/Patient Relationship

A priest who has not acquired the virtue of religion is an unsightly person. But how can today's secular doctor be expected to cultivate the virtue of religion without gross hypocrisy? Hippocratic and Galenic doctors were not religious in the ordinary sense of believing in a transcendent personal God who intervened in the lives of individuals and communities of people. Galen and his Hippocratic predecessors were the scientists of their day and indeed, would have to be called physicalists or materialists, rather than believers in a spiritual reality. And yet, they were religious and indeed advocated the virtue of religion in the sense of reverential awe in the presence of a "transcendent other."

The "other"—the "transcendent," the *quid divinum* for them was something which only the doctor encountered in the body of those whom he treated. The body for Galen, was a branch or sprout of nature (*physis*) which was god. The gods and nature were one and the same. All the essential roles of God as Transcendent Other, Hippocratic and later Galenic doctors attributed to nature from which the human body sprouted. Nature was both *tremendum* (causing one to tremble) and *fascinans* (fascinating, seductive). The body was *tremendum*, for example, when it decreed death for a patient or was incurable. It was *fascinans* and seductive when it permitted the doctor to catch a glimpse of an inherent wisdom, admirable and beautiful both in form and function.[12]

The body for Galen and his Hippocratic predecessors was the visible form of a divine nature (*physis*). As such, the body was sacred. Physicians who knew the body and worked with the body were expected to respond in a way appropriate to the reality which was encountered, and the appropriate response to an encounter with the sacred is the virtue of religion. The body, for pagan doctors, was the supreme epiphany of divine nature. Without being believers in the Greek pantheon, doctors were nevertheless expected to be religious and to develop religious virtues. Doctors, like the rest of us in contemporary America, show a religious reverence toward the dead body. We all dress up and adopt religious attitudes when a friend dies and is laid out. But somehow, we have forgotten this tradition regarding the living body. Historically, however, there was a religious dimension in the doctor/patient encounter which grounded the doctor's virtue of religion.

Even in today's doctor/patient relationship, there is a religious dimension in the sense that both doctors and patients hold beliefs about life and death. The science of medicine covers some dimensions of the doctor's life and medical practice, but lived reality is far too complex to be subsumed under any scientific paradigm, or directed strictly by scientific norms. In that sense, modern doctors are as religious as their Hippocratic predecessors were. They have to be. In fact, the most committed and convinced scientists are the strongest "religious" believers. First they believe in their science and then usually in all kinds of other propositions about life, politics, religion, etc., which can never be considered scientifically proven.

Patients, too, are believers. Their beliefs may come from traditional sources like Christianity or Judaism, or from more recent "religions" like Secular Individualism, Americanism, Humanism or Capitalism. But the fact is that both in doctors and in their patients, one will find non-scientific beliefs which stand at the center of who they are as persons. It is not required that every doctor/patient contact touch these deeper belief dimensions of personality, but there are times when ignoring these amounts to abandonment of the patient. Illness, especially serious illness, will call up every patient's belief system. Sometimes his or her belief system may be adequate to handle what is happening, but not always. A particular patient may be struggling to make some sense out of illness, and the doctor may be the only person who can help. Sometimes, at least, even secular doctors are forced to confront the deeper religious dimension of life.

Death and the Religious Dimension of Medicine

The religious dimension of the medical practice tends to be intensified by the doctor's constant contact with death. Historically, religion originated in consciousness of death, and for that reason, we find religion appearing at the earliest point of man's emergence from animal life. Nothing fixes human attention upon the ultimate questions and the possibility of "something more" than a reality so radically contigent. The frightful event of death, from which most human beings flee in order to live free from anxiety, the doctor can neither flee from nor repress for long. If doctors assist (stand close by) their patients in death, they cannot help but recognize their own eventual plight, and consequently, cannot help but pose for themselves all the questions about the meaning of life which we call "religious." Moral principles and medical codes reveal religious roots, and contemporary medical practice also has religious dimensions.

Because human beings are essentially religious animals and because religious issues are posited with particular urgency at the time of death, patients who are dying have special needs. Professionals other than doctors (e.g., clergy), may be primarily concerned with these needs, but many patients still look to the doctor for help at this difficult time. It is the doctor who, by obligation, discloses to the patient the truth about the time of death. And patients look to the doctor for assurance regarding some of their worst fears about death: dying in pain, lingering, choking, being abandoned, etc.

Because of the special affective relationship between the doctor and patient, it is not unusual that patients look to doctors for help of a spiritual sort.[13] No one knows how to die, but doctors at least have seen enough dying to know something about better and worse ways of dying. If the patient has developed a positive "transference" relationship with the physician, it is even more likely that he or she will expect the doctor to help with religious needs. Some patients specifically ask for help of this sort; others will be less forthcoming, but indicate in subtler ways their need. Doctors can meet certain spiritual needs of their patients only if they have developed a genuine religiosity.[14]

Ministering to the Dying

The writings of Dr. Elizabeth Kubler-Ross about death and dying have been turned into dogmas by some people. In fact, a new corps of "professionals" has emerged intent on making sure that every patient passes through each of the Kubler-Ross stages of dying in the appropriate order. Presumably, only they are prepared to meet the needs of the dying patient, and a new "profession" has come into being, a sort of secular, psychological priesthood.

But patients die in all kinds of ways and in many different psychological states, and new "secular priests" for the dying process ordinarily are not needed. The doctor who is sensitive to all of the dimensions of his patient's needs may be the best person to accompany a patient through the dying process. Patients who lived without religion will likely die without benefit of clergy. But since most people have "religious" needs at this time, the doctor may be the most indicated professional to help. If called upon for this kind of help, the doctor may want to be prepared to talk with patients about ultimate things. Doctors should not relegate their own priestly functions to others.

The last thing that any patient needs is to be assaulted at the time of death either by religious persons or their new secular counterparts. But doctors who are sensitive and respectful of religious differences can help patients with religious needs. The help that is called for at this delicate time is a response to what the patient needs and is not dictated by the doctor's particular religious tradition. Religious help for a dying patient, like all of the other help which a doctor provides, has to be dictated by what the patient needs and asks for. Attempts to convert patients or to "save" them on their deathbeds, or to make sure that they go through all the stages of dying, are out of place. But it would not be out of place for the doctor who understands the needs of his patients to share some thoughts about death if the patient is troubled by religious issues and wants help.

The Struggle with Despair and Dying

The most troublesome religious issue at the time of death is despair. Despair is painful because it is the nature of human beings to hope. Like all higher animals, human persons are alert to danger: they are "on guard." Future-oriented acts are grounded in man's animal biology and so it is not incorrect to say that we are naturally hopeful. As human animals, our biological orientation towards future good becomes transformed into *pro-jects* (literally to throw forward). Because of intelligence and imagination, we can look toward the future even when biological possibilities are fading in a dying process. Human orientation toward the "not yet," in the sense of possibility beyond this life, grounds one type of human religiosity. Human beings, in fact, must choose from among many imagined possibilities, including the God possibility. We are distinct from all other animals, because we invent our futures rather than simply adjust to present possibilities dictated by nature. Hope is rooted in biology, but we are carried beyond biology by our humanness.

Because human intelligence and imagination carry us beyond secure and fixed possibilities, in human hope there is a danger of failure or loss. The other side of human hope is human despair (literally, *des espoir*: without hope). Humans can increase natural hopeful sentiments with the use of drugs like alcohol, and hope is more intense at certain ages than at others. Some drunks are full of hope, and young people may be, too. The inflated hopes of the drunkard are transitory and quickly shrink into the next day's despair. Young people can also swing from great hope to terrible despair over issues which, for the more mature, merit neither reaction. Hope and despair rise and fall during the middle years, on the basis of projects initiated and projects failed. But toward the end of life, there are fewer projects to instill hope. Then the future narrows, expectations diminish, and even past projects which carried so much hope often appear as failures. If hope is built into the very animal structure of man, then despair, too, is part of who we are. As the human projects which characterized and indeed constituted a human life become impossible, persons naturally suffer despair.

Because despair is so painful and so frequently part of the dying process, it is not too much to say that it falls within the scope of a doctor's ministrations. Each physical loss causes a certain amount of despair, and when physical disintegration slips beyond medical help, despair may be severe. When a human being can no longer expect remedy and can look forward with certainty only to death, who can cope? What can provide hope when human powers and medicine's art are spent? Only what is beyond nature. At the time of death, patients either hope for a future good, or they have to find the courage to die in despair. With either final struggle, patients may need the doctor's help.

At the point of death, human beings become religious, at least in the extended understanding of this term. The patient either believes that there is something more or that there is nothing more. In either case, patients move to a level of belief because neither response is dictated by scientific evidence. Atheism, in the sense of embracing despair, and theism, as an embracing of hope in a future good, are both religious "stands." Proof runs out at this point and opens up space for a leap of faith. For this reason, it makes sense to speak of a religious dimension to the doctor/patient relationship and to include a virtue of religion among those others which help a physician to become a good doctor.

For the atheist, doctors can be understanding and assist (stand close by) so that the patient does not die alone. For the patient whose hope transforms the losses associated with death into expectations of future good, the doctor's helping role may pass to others, such as clergy and family. But for the many modern persons of our secular society who are neither true atheists nor persons practicing religion, the doctor may be the only source of help during a period of painful doubt. Some doctors, themselves secular persons, feel helpless in the face of death and regularly flee to more medically hopeful cases. But doctors who aspire to be good by trying to meet all the patient's needs have to reconsider what, to a contemporary secular physician, may seem preposterous: i.e., a joining of medicine and religion; requiring of a doctor the virtue of religion; accepting the idea of doctor as priest.

The Virtue of Religion for Doctors

Doctors will always be expected to be different from other professionals, and the difference will be traceable to a priestly dimension of the doctor/patient relationship. Disappointment and a feeling of betrayal will always result when doctors act just like everyone else. If there is a priestly dimension to doctoring, then it is reasonable to suggest doctors strive to develop the virtue of religion. The worst of all situations would be to adopt a false and pretentious priestliness to cover up self-serving practices. The term, religion, refers to a virtue which disposes in the very opposite direction.

Traditionally, the virtue of religion referred to an inner willingness to offer oneself in the service of God. For the believing doctor, that traditional understanding still applies. Using an expanded understanding of the objective meaning of religion (to refer to whatever is included under deep beliefs), we can expand the meaning of religion as virtue to apply to doctors who do not think of themselves as religious in a traditional sense. A doctor's religion in this expanded sense would require reflection on the awesome dimensions of his work; recognition of what is "transcendent" in the patient (the mystery of human life); and commitment to serving patients struggling with life's meaning.

The doctor's subjective virtue of religion would add a sense of reverence to his or her helping medical acts. It would invoke a consciously cultivated resistance to treating patients routinely or impersonally. For the Christian doctor, the virtue of religion would mean treating the patient as Christ; for a Jewish doctor, recognizing the patient as a child of God; for a secular doctor, religion could be the religion of Galen and Hippocrates, for whom contact with the marvelous systems of the body was a contact with a *quid divinum*. The "divine" would be revealed in the body which decrees health and at some point, death. So inevitable is the decree that in the dying process the doctor can only bow, adopt a reverential attitude and be willing to help.

Besides providing a tone of piety toward the patient, the virtue of religion would dispose doctors to attend to the patient's religious needs, no matter how they manifest themselves. A doctor's virtue of religion is related to beneficence, as is the case with all of the other virtues. It also disposes the doctor to meet patient needs. Religion is always "other-directed" and in the case of a doctor's religiousness, the "other" is the patient.

There has always been a religious and priestly dimension to medical practice, and a danger will always exist that medical religiousness may become self-serving rather than patient serving. The virtue of religion disposes a doctor to practice a patient-centered medicine, and care must be taken lest medical religion become corrupted into an idolatrous ideology. Instead of permitting a person to understand, ideology clouds the truth about reality, our own and the others'. Because they are under attack from many sides, the medical profession and individual doctors could turn selfish interests into an ideology that puts the doctor at the center of concern instead of the patient. If this happens, the patient's situation will slide farther and farther from view. The virtue of religion is a defense against such a distortion.

The virtue of religion not only keeps the "Transcendent Other" in first place, but disposes toward service of the "other" rather than oneself. It keeps doctors from confusing themselves with God, and from falling into the temptation of moral self-righteousness. It is the reality of God that keeps creatures aware of "their place" and of who is really holy. The virtue of religion is the habit of keeping this order straight. Not only are human beings of power and privilege inclined to confuse themselves with God, but also to confuse their interest with moral right. The defense of power and privilege inevitably takes on a phony religious tone—and the true virtue of religion would guard against this false religiosity.

Historically, ethical values and principles have been rooted in religious belief, and this is certainly true of Western ethics. The Ten Commandments have been the standards of both individual and social morality in the West, and these norms rest on a claim of God's miraculous intervention in history. Ethics is not reducible to religion, nor religion to ethics, but ethics opens up to religion both as its source and as its final fulfillment. The Western value system, including ethical values incorporated into lived behavior through virtues and character, is both grounded in religion and requires a belief commitment. The good doctor, like any good person, must be religious in the sense of placing himself or herself in the service of the "other" rather than the self.

Neither self will, nor self-creation, nor self-righteousness can be a foundation for a medical ethics.

The sense of being indebted to the "Other," and the corresponding disposition to reverence by helping in all of the ways the "other" needs help is what the virtue of religion is all about for doctors. This virtue permeates the Hippocratic, as well as the Western medical tradition. The good doctor is conscious of what is owed to "others." Being religious means being aware of a debt and being disposed to repay it.

Notes

1. Gracia-Guillen, Diego, "Profession o Sacerdocio? Propuestas para un debate etico sobre la profesion medica," *Jano*, Madrid, 1983. I studied History of Medicine with my friend Diego Gracia in Madrid during 1987 and am endebted to him for much of the material in this chapter.

2. *Deuteronomy*, Chapter 17:8-13.

3. *Leviticus*, Chapters 13, 14, 15.

4. *Leviticus*, Chapter 21:16-22.

5. Hippocrates, *Hippocratic Oath*, Loeb Classical Library, vol. I, (Cambridge, MA: Harvard University Press), 1962. Translation mine.

6. Hippocrates, *The Law*, Loeb Classical Library, vol. II, (Cambridge, MA: Harvard University Press), 1962, p. 265.

7. Hippocrates, *The Physician*, Loeb Classical Library, vol. II, (Cambridge, MA: Harvard University Press)., 1962, pp. 311, 312.

8. The whole text of the Hippocratic writing *Decorum*, witnesses to the many aspects of the good physician's character—both the real virtues and the proper appearances. Hippocrates, *Decorum*, Loeb Classical Library, vol. II, (Cambridge, MA: Harvard University Press), 1962, pp. 279-301.

9. Bullough, V.L., *The Development of Medicine as a Profession: The Contribution of the Medieval University to Modern Medicine*, (New York: S. Karger), 1960.

10. Clark, G.A., *History of the Royal College of Physicians of London*, vol. I, (Oxford: Clevendon Press), 1964.

11. Ibid.

12. Lain Entralgo, Pedro, *Historia de la Medicina*, (Madrid: Salvat), 1985, p. 71.

13. Eric Cassell tells a story about a modern woman who no longer has any religious faith and yet is afraid of death. She says, "For me, the doctor is now God. Now there is only the

doctor to protect me." Cassell, E.J., *The Healer's Art: A New Approach to the Doctor-Patient Relationship.* (Baltimore: Penguin), 1979, p. 182.

14. There are programs available to nurses which are aimed at developing their spirituality and sensitizing them to meet the spiritual needs of patients. RISEN, (Re-Investigating Spirituality and Ethics in Nursing), which combines ethical and spiritual development for nurses, is based at the Catholic Health Association of Wisconsin. To my knowledge, no such formalized program exists for doctors, but the Catholic Physician's Guild and the *Linacre Quarterly* do address the religion-medicine relationship.

Part II

Justifying Character and Virtue in Medical Ethics

8.

American Medical Ethics and Loss of Concern for Ethical Self

There may be more pluralistic nations than the United States, but not many. As far as morality is concerned, there are almost as many different ways of judging right from wrong as there are individual Americans. With such diversity, the law has become our only unifying standard. Right and wrong is reduced to what is or is not against the law, and law has come to be the social institution to which Americans look for resolution of ethical disputes. If resolution of disputes rather than concern for character becomes the central concern of medical ethics as well as law, then fact clarifications and the creation of concrete action guides become the essential activities. All other considerations are either ignored or denied relevance.

The number of lawyers and lawsuits shows the extent to which the law functions in America as a moral arbitrator. In fact, the law sets standards even for how professional ethicists work. Ethics becomes a decision-making methodology that is a conscious or unconscious imitation of the law. In law court, first the facts that bear on a dispute are marshalled and the issue to be decided is defined. Once the preliminary fact-gathering and clarification are completed, other judicial decisions which serve as standards (precedents) are identified. Finally, a judgment is rendered by applying the precedent to the facts. In the law, facts plus standards produce specific, concrete judgments.

Ethics practiced by most American ethicists operates in much the same way. Robert M. Veatch, a major player on the American medical ethics scene, puts the process for coming to ethical decisions in medicine into a simple syllogistic form. "If conditions A, B, C, D, E and F exist, then based on evaluative framework X, Y, Z, one might do M. Conditions A, B, C, D, E and F exist. Therefore, one ought to do M."[1] The evaluative framework which Veatch has in mind is not law, but the process for arriving at decisions is the same. Because of the many different forms of evaluative frameworks used by Americans, Veatch concludes that the doctor's own standards of evaluation, have no priority over anyone else's. He wants to bring more equality into the doctor/patient relationship.

Most medical ethicists have degrees in philosophy, and therefore are not unsophisticated in their understanding of the decision-making process. The application of a legal precedent may be quite literal and even somewhat mechanical, but this is not so in clinical cases centering on ethics. The very identification of relevant facts, as well as their assessment, depends upon a person's framework of ethical beliefs and value assumptions. In ethics, it is never a question of simply applying a universally recognized standard to an agreed upon set of facts to get the one and only right or wrong thing to do. In a clinical setting, there will be different right and wrong responses depending upon the evaluator's understanding of facts and his or her beliefs about the most relevant ethical guides. And yet, the process by which ethical decisions are made in

American hospitals is not substantially different from the legal process. In law, as well as in American style medical ethics, the understanding of what ethics is all about aspires to the pragmatic goal of arriving at concrete norms which work out in practice and are legally defensible.

Another major figure in American medical ethics is Tom Beauchamp.[2] Like Robert Veatch, he is on the staff at the Kennedy Institute at Georgetown University. Ethics for Beauchamp is about actions and action guides. Each culture develops its own ethical behaviors and transmits them from generation to generation. Essentially and fundamentally, ethics is about rules of behavior, which along with customs and rules of other sorts, make up a social fabric. Ethics as customs is something objective and endures beyond the lifespan of individual members of society. Like language, ethics for Beauchamp is "out there" when individuals come on the scene, and it endures beyond their demise.

Ethicists reflect on these objective institutions and try to introduce clarity and precision to ethical discussions. They try to organize the social practices and moral customs into a coherent and unified system, sometimes supporting existing ethical practice and at other times challenging it. In effect, they attempt to justify a certain organization of rules and practices, by arguments which rely heavily on abstract action-guides called principles. Ethics, for Beauchamp, is not different from what the ancients would have referred to as technical knowledge. There are general action guides and narrow rules of behavior which medical professionals can learn to apply adroitly to concrete moral difficulties. The behaviors are out there in the public domain, and if a physician receives good training in logic, he or she can clarify behavior dilemmas and arrive at publicly defensible decisions. Ethics is knowledge of means to this end. For Tom Beauchamp and most American medical ethicists, the task of the ethicist is to disentangle the confusion in which medical ethics cases are embedded. Once a case under consideration is clarified, and the principles or action guides which themselves have to be disentangled from the same social fabric, are applied, we can arrive at right decisions.

Historically, these views of ethics parallel those of the Sophists who also construed ethics in terms of rules and technical knowledge. Aristotle and Plato opposed this understanding. They did not deny the relevance for ethics as concrete rules and technical knowledge for coming to correct decisions about human affairs, but thought such an understanding was too narrow. Plato thought that ethics was also about the way people are, or about *being* as well as *doing*. More than action guides and technical skills in applying them, ethics is also about reflection on the quality of persons who act, and about ways to improve the attitudes and dispositions of persons. In this other sense, ethics is less technical, but not simply a matter of personal taste either. It is both personal and objective.

American medical ethicists, who focus on the technical dimensions of decision-making, have made important contributions. Beauchamp and Veatch, for example, are scholars with international reputations that are well deserved. While they go about their business in medical ethics, however, they are also becoming certain types of persons. And each brought a well developed character structure to his academic work in ethics. The same is true for practicing doctors and lawyers. The question is whether this is important or whether the traditional concern of ethics for the acting person deserves a place in modern medical ethics. Other important medical ethicists like William F. May[3] and Renee Fox[4] think that character and virtue definitely belong in medical ethics. Theirs is not a criticism of what is being done with objective rules and standards, but rather a suggestion that the perspective be broadened to include personal attitudes, dispositions and habits, as well as actions, rules and principles.

The ethical tradition of Aristotle and Plato was never abandoned in religious ethics. In Catholic ethics, for example, a distinction was always made between the *right* and the *good*. Terms like right and wrong refer to characteristics of an action. Right actions are those which conform to moral standards and to an objective moral order. In this tradition, the moral order is grounded in the human person and the human community. What promotes the person and community is right; what destroys or diminishes either is wrong. The terms good and bad, however, refer to a person's intentions, attitudes and character. A good person can do a wrong thing without becoming bad, and a bad person can occasionally do a right act.

American medical ethics has been more concerned with the right than with the good. It has been concerned with the objective dimensions and has concentrated on finding solutions to complex problems. Very little consideration has been given to the character or virtues appropriate to a good doctor.[5]

To insist on a place for character in medical ehtics is to say that the original meaning of *ethos* (the inner self) is relevant to what goes on in medicine. Individual acts, chosen and repeated, obviously have an effect on the kind of person one becomes. By individual acts of selfless caring for the sick, a doctor becomes a caring self. By repeated just acts, he makes himself just. Acts follow one upon another, but gradually they leave something permanent in their wake. That something is a reality which gives unity to acts and keeps life from being a disconnected chaos of behaviors. Doctors, like everyone else, or perhaps more so than others, develop certain attitudes, dispositions and character traits. Medical ethics, it seems, should be concerned with this fact.

An American commission on the teaching of bioethics worked for four years[6] to examine the goals, problems and future of bioethics teaching. This group listed the following goals for medical ethics education: 1) to identify and define moral issues in a bio-medical context, 2) to develop strategies for analyzing moral problems in medicine, 3) to relate principles to specific issues and cases, 4) to train a small group for careers in bioethics. The same exclusive concern with the objective dimensions of ethics can be seen in a later report on medical ethics teaching in American medical schools.[7] An update on the teaching of medical ethcs in medical schools showed the same focus on objective features as the earlier report and explicitly excluded issues of character from consideration.[8]

American medical ethics reflects a high degree of intelligent manipulation of the external aspects of ethics. Nowhere else are problems laid out and analyzed so precisely. An effort is made to understand a dilemma from every perspective, and to weigh risks and benefits before coming to any decision. This act analysis *par excellence* both enriches and impoverishes the ethical enterprise in medicine. The impoverishment derives from ignoring the person who acts: the *ethos* of the doctor who treats patients. Kant, in a sense, took for granted the objective content of moral behavior, assuming that everyone knew and accepted Christian standards of right behavior. American medical ethicists in the Kantian tradition, along with their utilitarian colleagues, take the subjective dimension for granted. Ethics is practiced by medical ethicists as if neither their own characters nor the character of the physician had anything to do with the enterprise.

More than one reason can be found for this one-sidedness. We already mentioned the influence of language. The fact that our word "ethics" carries more of the Latin meaning of *mos moris* (i.e. behavior) certainly plays a role. Our language turns reflection toward behavior considerations. Then, too, although the inner being or character of a person is as real as the person's acts, it is a much subtler reality, and consequently is more difficult to analyze and to work with. Finally, medical ethics in the West was for centuries linked to Catholic moral theology which was heavily oriented toward act analysis.[9]

Long before bioethics became the popular discipline that it is today, medical ethics was a standard subject in seminaries. The concerns in those courses were issues of birth and death, and the focus was on how to analyze cases which people brought to the priest. The pre-Vatican II focus on the Sacrament of Penance dictated the flavor and direction of moral theological reflection. Confessors had to make quick judgments on cases because there was usually a long line waiting outside. There was little time for considerations of character. It was the objective feature of the case at hand which required attention, analysis, and finally, judgment about degree of culpability. One aspect of Catholic ethics is act analysis and so too is the secular medical ethics which followed in its footsteps.

Concern about the character and inner being of the person survived in Catholic thought primarily in Ascetic theology and spiritual direction, but it did not find a place in secular medical ethics.[10]

In another sense, the act analysis orientation of American medical ethics merely reflects the loss of concern about inner being and character in contemporary American culture. Modern Americans identify with science and technology, to the point of looking at their own lives through these narrow perspectives. What science identifies as real is what is physical and measurable. Acts, therefore, are real, but not a person's character or inner self. These latter are "unreal," or "mystical," or "philosophical nonsense," and even a mention of such topics in some company today would likely be greeted with a condescending look of disbelief. Genetics, environmental signals, organs, tissues, neurons, nueronal transmitters, hormones: this is what human life is all about. A sense of inner self which is free to respond to the outside as possiblity and to create itself is out of place in this point of view.

The machines which surround contemporary persons and with which their lives are so immersed also have an influence. They dictate the way we think of ourselves. Production quotas and work routines push people toward self-forgetfulness. Life itself is experienced as a machine: a production center moved by outside factors. Leisure, which once was time for self-remembering, has become a form of self-forgetting (not reading and reflection, but distractions and activities). The fact that the self is forgotten in ethics is not too difficult to understand. In some sense, both modern ethics and modern American medical ethics reflect contemporary life.

Cognitive frameworks and styles of reflection follow from cultural and disciplinary identification, and this means persons working in an American cultural context tend to collapse character considerations into privacy concerns. This one widely accepted moral value grounds the ethical principles of autonomy and the sanctity of life. It also grounds the lists of ethical and legal rights which each person can claim against individual others or against society. Among these are the "right" to decide how each will live to attain maximum individual well-being.

American rights tend to be negative ones in the sense that persons may not be interfered with in the pursuit of individual projects as long as the rights of others are not violated. This is as close as mainline medical ethics comes to character consideration.

The emphasis on privacy and negative individual rights also explains the great importance given to the rules and norms of informed consent. Literature on this one topic in American medical ethics is enormous. Hefty volumes have recently been written by Tom Beauchamp and Paul Applebaum,[11] and new books are added every year. The underlying asumption throughout this literature is that the doctor/patient relationship is one between two autonomous individuals, one of whom is disadvantaged by the doctor's power and needs protection lest harm occur in the form of not being able to carry out wishes.

There is, however, more to the doctor/patient relationship than two autonomous individuals exercising their freedom. The two persons are either well or poorly developed characters, and the ethical quality of this important relationship depends heavily on qualities of character. Whether or not the doctor/patient relationship qualifies as ethical, humane, helpful, respectful, etc., has to do with many personal characteristics which fall outside informed consent directives. Informed consent literature pays close attention to the things a doctor must disclose in order that the autonomous patient can make an informed choice. But whether or not the patient is able to choose freely also depends upon whether truthful relevant information is discerned and how it is communicated. For this, the physician's character is crucial.

The backgrounds of practicing bioethicists as well as the peculiar concerns of American culture have obscured the importance of character and virtue in medical ethics. And yet, these ethical categories cannot constitute the heart and soul of a medical ethical tradition for centuries, and then suddenly lose all relevance. Finding a place for their discussion is difficult, however, without some rethinking of the foundations of medical ethics. As things presently stand, character and virtue fall outside the narrow paradigm in which medical ethical discussion occurs. Bio-ethicists in America have their own way of defining what a legitimate bio-ethical concern is. Verifiable facts, logical arguments, methodological rules and privacy concerns are central. Character is not a clear enough concept, not objective enough, not precise enough to fit this model.

Another way to speak of the American medical ethics enterprise is to say that it is dominated by abstract principles. Because bio-ethicists are usually philosophers, they know that the principles of autonomy, beneficence and justice depend upon philosophical assumptions about life which ultimately are grounded in beliefs. And yet the principles which dominate medical ethical thinking are consciously or unconsciously considered to be out there, and if not taken for granted, they are taken to be objectively correct. Teaching a course in bio-ethics at a foreign medical school, any person quickly realizes that American principles, values, and beliefs are far from universal. Not moving outside the States, one can easily be led to believe that American philosophy, derived from its utilitarian and Kantian beliefs, and its preoccupation with methodology and pragmatic norms, is all there is to medical ethics. A scientific assumption on the part of many physicians is very compatable with a similar positivism operating in American medical ethics.

In this context, character considerations and virtue appropriate to physicians have little relevance, and indeed, the topics may be treated with scorn. The very words, character and virtue, have a religious ring to the secular thinker, which is reason enough to consider them out of place. To be seriously considered, these terms would have to be "laundered" and "operationalized." Consequently, bio-ethics moves ahead with its orientation toward problem solving, privacy concerns and the construction of concrete norms that a pluralist society can live with. The pressing nature of more and more ethical problems forces attention to fact clarification and policy making, and leaves little time for other dimensions. As bio-ethics with such a reduced and narrowed foundation expands, character, virtue and a host of other ethical dimensions of medical practice fade further and further from view. There is no room for what used to be called "Habits of the Heart."

Notes

1. Veatch, Robert M., "Lay Medical Ethics," *Journal of Medicine and Philosophy*, 10, February, 1985.

2. Beauchamp, Thomas, *Case Studies in Business, Society, and Ethics*, (Englewood Cliffs, NJ: Prentice Hall), 1983. See also, Tom Beauchamp and James F. Children, *Principles of Biomedical Ethics*, (New York: Oxford University Press), 1983; and Tom Beauchamp and Ruth Faden, (eds.), *Ethical Issues in Social Science Research*, (Baltimore: Johns Hopkins University Press), 1982.

3. May, William F., *The Physician's Covenant*, (London: Westminster Press), 1983.

4. Fox, Renee C., *Essays in Medical Sociology*, (New York: Wilen), 1979.

5. Stanley Hauerwas is an exception to this rule. He has written several important books on character and has made substantial contributions to Medical Ethics literature. Cf. *A Community of Character*, (Notre Dame, IN: University of Notre Dame Press), 1981, and, *The Peaceable Kingdom*, (University of Notre Dame Press), 1983. Other works include Hauerwas, Stanley, *Character and the Christian Life: A Study in Theological Ethics*, (San Antonio: Trinity University Press), 1985; Hauerwas, Stanley, *Suffering Presence: Theological Reflections on Medicine, the Mentally Handicapped and the Church*. (University of Notre Dame Press), 1986; and Hauerwas, Stanley, *Vision and Virtue: Essays in Christian Ethical Reflection*, (University of Notre Dame Press), 1981.

6. Teaching of Bioethics: *Report of the Commission on the Teaching of Bioethics*, (Hastings on the Hudson, NY: Institute of Society, Ethics, and Life Sciences), 1976.

7. Veatch, Robert M. and Sharmon Sollitto, "Medical Ethics Teaching," *Journal of the American Medical Association*, Vol. 235, No. 10, March 8, 1976.

8. Culver, Charles M., et.al., "Basic Curricular Goals in Medical Ethics," *New England Journal of Medicine*, Vol. 312, No. 4, 1985.

9. Catholic moral theology especially was concerned with deciding which acts were sins and which were not. One sees this act emphasis in the pioneering work of 20th century Jesuit thinkers like Ford, Kelly, Healy, McCormick, McFadden, and O'Donnell. The work of these Irish-American Jesuits continues a Catholic tradition that goes back many centuries to Spaniards like Suarez, Soto, and de Victoria.

10. Today's secular version of the spiritual director is the psycho-analytically oriented therapist. Not without some reason then, does Thomas Szasz make the point again and again in his books on psychiatry that the therapist is more priest or ethical counselor than doctor.

11. Applebaum, Paul; Litz, Charles; and Alan Meisel, *Informed Consent, Legal Theory, and Clinical Practice*, (New York: Oxford University Press), 1987. See also, Faden, Ruth and Thomas Beauchamp, *A History and Theory of Informed Consent*, (New York: Oxford University Press), 1986.

9.

Getting in Touch with the Ethical Self

If there is more to ethics than act analysis and norm development, and if American medical ethics would be enriched by a more adequate theoretical base, which included consideration of character and the acting person, then a first step would have to be clarification of what character or ethical self means. For modern Americans it is at best an ambiguous notion. Perhaps the best way to understand it is to do a simple reflection on personal experience.

It is not difficult for contemporary persons to recognize that their lives are absorbed in external activities. The experience of an inner self in danger of being lost in things and senseless acts is actually quite a common one. People then usually try to reverse this process by searching for a stronger or deeper self through therapy or meditation. But a simple examination of conscience, which can take place even during an unguarded few moments in a busy schedule can also put a person into contact with the inner self. Unlike religious meditation, self-remembering has no holy object, nor does it require a sacred place. It is simply being alone with one's self.

A doctor, for example, might begin by examining the behaviors and attitudes which reflect his inner self. Am I helpful? sincere? respectful to patients? dishonest? authentic? evasive? resentful? The inner ethos which a person finds in meditation or self-examination is neither a purely psychic disposition, nor the effect of an outside environment. The *ethos* is what persons make of their psychic disposition and the circumstances in which they find themselves. The inner self is personality, looked at in terms of ethical categories. Character is another word for the same reality.

I can contact my inner self, and I can choose to give my character a certain direction. The self as chosen is the meaning of *ethos* or character. It is my way of being related to the world and other people, and it expresses itself in chosen attitudes and patterns of behavior. Not only do I judge this or that action, but I judge my very self. I might even direct certain admonitions to my inner self, like: "be more considerate," "let the other person be," "don't be so serious," "life is a gift—be thankful for it." The character which I discover and try to improve is the ethical structure of my personality.

Although character considerations are absent from medical ethics, American style, they have not disappeared from ordinary language. People talk about character types with commonly used terms like yuppie, hippie, jock, social butterfly, academic, religious, etc. These terms refer to certain persons' way of being, especially to their ways of responding to other people and to the world around them. Sometimes words like *personality* or *identity* will be used to refer to ethical self or character, but in most contexts they have a predominately psychological flavor. Character considerations, then, are absent neither from ordinary people's concerns nor from ordinary language. The word *character* is frequently used and refers to good character in the sense of having principles and sticking to them, risking unpopularity to do what's right, having courage of convictions, being fair, being unselfish, being able to rebound from a failure, etc. Integrity, like character, has strong ethical overtones, and both terms have much to do with intention and good will.

What one does not find in ordinary language and among the issues ordinary people think about is a theory of character. For that we have to look to moral philosophers and theologians. Soren Kierkegaard is the philosopher par excellence of ethical character.[1] For him, the inner self paradoxically is and comes to be in acts of self-choice joined to total commitment. He talks about more mystical routes to the apprehension of one's inner ethical self than simply examining one's conscience. He speaks of *Der Augenblick,* literally the blink of an eye in which one's *ethos* or inner ethical being becomes present to consciousness. In an instant, a character type which he calls "the aesthete" sees his inner self as uncommitted, superficial, narcissistic and dissipated in every passing moment. *Ethos* as inner ethical being for Kierkegaard is revealed in a privileged insight. We do not consciously seek out the revelation as in an examination of conscience, but rather all of a sudden (*der Augenblick*), there it is. And there we are. Not inconsistently, Kierkegaard held that contemporary man is more in need of this revelation than persons in other ages. Self forgetting must be overcome before a person can come into contact with his or her character.

Revelation of one's own *ethos* for Kierkegaard is a precondition for the necessary choice of a certain self that makes a person ethical. First, we have to see the inner self: we have to come to know ourselves. Then, we can set out to form or reform this self by a conscious choice. We can choose the self as it is—or we can choose a new self in the sense of a new ethical being committed to values beyond narcissism and convenience. This new inner self—which Kierkegaard calls an ethical self— is first and foremost the inner being which in one sense we already are, but in a fuller sense, a new reality which we bring into being by serious choice. The ethical self is the foundation of ethics in the sense that specific acts are its expression. The resentful person, for example, is just one example of an inner self which expresses itself in actions and patterns. The bigot, the miser, the lover, and all the above mentioned more modern types (hippies, yuppies, etc.) are other possibilities. The "good doctor" also refers to a certain type of self and a particular way of being which expresses itself in countless acts that are important in medicine but have no place in medical ethics.

Kierkegaard would be appalled by a medical ethics which ignored the doctor's character, because for him, ethics is character. He stands at the opposite pole from present day American medical ethics, and it may be interesting to listen to this distinctive personality who not only thought about character, but had one. "Morality is character, character is that which is engraved (καρασσοω); but the sand and the sea have no character and neither has abstract intelligence, for character is really inwardness."[2]

Death is another revealer of *ethos*. We are all familiar with the reports of persons who have had close calls with death. "My life passed before my eyes" is one way of talking about the experience. Others talk about "seeing life in its totality" or "seeing one's inner self." Tolstoy, in the story *The Death of Ivan Illich*,[3] gives us a marvelous account of self-perception, slowed down over the period of sickness. Not in an instant or an *Augenblick*, but gradually, Ivan caught a glimpse of the person he had been, his *ethos*, and set out in his last days to forge a different, more authentic self. He saw the structure of his former self and rejected it for a more honest way of being. His new inner ethical being, in turn, changed Ivan's way of being with others in the world. The old foundation of action was replaced by a new one. The new *ethos* was the final Ivan Illich, and the act of choice which brought it into being was the most important ethical event of his life. Something similar can be imagined with doctors who frequently experience death in sympathetic identification with their patients. These privileged moments can help a doctor to come into contact with the inner self.

Whether it is death that reveals, or a privileged *Augenblick*, or a mere prosaic systematic searching out of self through meditation, the point is that each person's *ethos* is an important ethical reality. And this fundamental ethical reality is a human creation. Using the language of theology, we can say that God creates human life in the sense of providing the raw materials of existence. Then, human beings create themselves in the sense of forging for themselves a self which was not determined to be but comes into being as a result of free decisions.

The second creation of an ethical inner being depends upon a total and permanent commitment to someone or something. At some point, a doctor, for example, decided upon a career in medicine, and that decision was accompanied by a commitment to be a certain type person. Not uncommonly, but paradoxically, that original moral commitment is lost in the course of medical training. But rarely is it totally destroyed. Something remains, and that something can be renewed. Some ethical failures in medicine derive from the doctor's never having been committed seriously to anyone or any ideal beyond his or her well-being. Far more commonly, ethical faults result from a weakening of an original commitment, and its associated ethical ideals. What comes into being by choice can be weakened by other choices and even lost by neglect.

The instant in which an ethical inner self comes into being does not end the creative process. Self-creation is initiated, but not finished, in an instant. *Ethos* is forged in the many tiny choices which follow a fundamental choice. Each successive moment, event, or situation, provides an opportunity for the creation to continue or for a slide backward toward aesthetic self-absorption. It is one thing to create an inner ethical self by self-choice; it is another thing to bring that creation to development.

Because each creation is different, there are many different types of character. In choosing to be a certain person, each person launches a drama, and no two "plays" are alike. Because maturing or perfecting one's character takes time, patience is required to become ethical. No one can force the circumstances which call for critical response of the inner self which in turn solidifies a character. On the other hand, we only have a certain limited time to carry out our ethical enterprise. Death fixes forever the *ethos* we have created.

Why Create a Self?

One option for the human person is not to choose or to choose not to create a self at all, but simply to live out one's empirical existence. We all find ourselves with a certain body, a set of dispositions, a particular family, and a certain socio-economic condition. The phrase, empirical existence, refers to this given with which each life finds itself. The physical given and the socio-cultural environment can dominate a life. Human beings, for instance, can simply respond to the many conditions which present themselves so as to maximize personal convenience and minimize inconvenience. "Taking care of number one" is an example of this and happens to constitute the conventional ethical wisdom of our American culture. And it is symbolized in the self-centered forms of therapy which provide spiritual direction for today's secular souls in search of salvation. And yet, serious philosophical anthropology (as opposed to pop psychology) assures us that following this "common wisdom" leads gradually to increasing isolation, then melancholy, and finally despair.[4]

Depression, which is so common today, apparently is despair about this or that event or circumstance. In fact, however, it is usually despair about oneself. The self can enter into despair about itself because empirical existence, or the given self, is meant to be the raw material of a chosen or created self and not a final product. By choosing to commit one's empirical existence to an ideal, empirical existence is given a new form. Some people, however, never make a self-creating choice. They confront life with the question, "What shall I do?" and answer, "I'll do whatever is required to preserve my empirical existence." Frequently, human beings try to save their lives (empirical existence) at the expense of their inner being or character. An inner self or created self never comes to be, and life without inner being gradually senses its radical deficiency. It is this deficiency which stands behind so much of the depression and despair characteristic of our times.

The person without a self becomes dispirited, and the root cause of this situation, according to Kierkegaard, is disobedience. The command that is disobeyed is: "A human being must become a self." Human beings must create an inner self by choosing to form life according to some ideal. The imperative, "Be yourself," means "Become someone;" "Create an inner being in the smithy of your soul." From the sophisticated reflections expressed in the Genesis stories (mistaken by Fundamentalists to be a scientific account of the origin of the cosmos), we learn that ethical failure comes from disobedience. The basic and most fundamental ethical failure is disobedience to the command which echoes in the structure of human being itself. "Doing what is right" or "becoming good" first of all means working to create one's own character.

Creating an *ethos* always involves commitment to a project. Human beings make themselves not out of nothing, but with the cooperation of both intelligence and freedom. Once an inner ethical being is created, human life becomes something more. It is given a new depth, a greater significance, and a reason for hope. None of this is immediately evident on the outside. The inner creation is never demonstrable by scientific criteria. But when it takes place, it makes all the difference in the way a person acts. It is like that mysterious moment when a seed breaks apart and sinks its roots. It happens in a moment, and yet it permits the moments which follow to have a unity, a direction and an inner consistency.

Ethos, obviously is not itself visible, but yet can be seen in attitudes of perseverance, or fidelity, or courage in times of stress. Despite slips and falls, character shows itself in a willingness to start again in the chosen direction. It becomes evident in the stands people take which cost dearly in terms of personal comfort. In rare occasions, the cost is total: the very sacrifice of empirical existence. Socrates showed his inner ethical being in the face of death. He could have escaped and did not. He made visible to his students a character without anger, hatred or resentment. All the drives and instincts of empirical existence had been reformed by his commitment to truth, his dedication to goodness and his belief in immortality. St. Thomas More is another person who shows us the influence of a chosen and re-chosen ethical being.[5] He is a man for all seasons because of the strength and unpretentiousness of his character. The lives of both men show clearly that the creation of an inner self has everything to do with ethics. In their cases, an objective analysis of acts alone would miss the most important of all ethical realities.

But if there are saints who show us an inner ethical being in ideal form, there are also lives which show us clearly the absence of an *ethos*, or a defective character. The *aesthete* is committed to never choosing a self, and to his or her own gratification. Other persons are opportunities for manipulation or seduction, but little else. Where empirical existence dominates, personal convenience reigns. Everyone has come across persons who may be fun to be with socially, but cannot be counted on for anything beyond chit-chat. These persons actually are not unethical; rather, they have not yet reached the ethical stage which comes to be only after commitment to someone or something beyond the empirical self. The self-centered, ego-centric personality is an example of defective or ethically undeveloped character. Some persons who run large institutions and make big money are just such moral cripples. Making money or being successful in America does not require an ethical development. In fact, ethics may be a real drawback.

Another interesting type of unethical character is the hypocrite. With the hypocrite there is a pretense of commitment to ideals or goals beyond personal pleasure and convenience, but under the slightest pretense, ideals are abandoned. Closely related to the hypocritical self is the role player who is whatever the outside circumstance dictates. The root problem in both cases is superficial character and subsequently deficient acts. The weak self of the hypocrite and the role player is capable of the worst imaginable evil actions. He, like the *aesthete*, will do almost anything to preserve empirical life. Missing from such an *ethos* is strength, steadfastness and freedom to do something with his life against the pressure of circumstance. Hannah Arendt, in her book on Adolf Eichmann, showed how enormous evil can originate from an ethically weak, indeed banal, *ethos*.[6]

Finally, we can understand the evil actions of persons who choose to create an unethical self. Rather than choosing a self committed to ideals and caring for being, humans are able to create an immoral *ethos*, committed to the distortion of ideals and the destruction of being. The very opposite of the saint is the evil character whose life is dominated by forms of death dealing behavior. Character in the sense of good character manifests itself in acts which affirm life, and bad character shows itself in acts of willful destructiveness. The good person builds the human by being committed to someone or something beyond self. The evil person sows hate and destruction.

Doctors in Western history have generally been considered good persons. Medical ethics was for centuries synonymous with character development, and historically, when doctors were challenged, they always used good ethical character and priestly virtue to justify their social position.[7] The same high standards of character development, as we have seen, were expected of doctors and priests.

Bio-ethicists can afford to ignore character considerations because good character is still assumed among medical professionals. Ordinarily doctors are good persons in the sense of honest and caring selves. The literature and tradition surrounding character building and the ways character traits are taught can be considered superfluous as long as there is no evidence of character failure among doctors. What may once have been true, however, cannot continue to be counted on. And even without pressures created by the loss of traditional ways of being a good doctor, there are reasons to take another look at what discussion of character might do to improve the ethical quality of modern medicine.

A commitment to be a doctor is usually a commitment to a higher form of ethical self. Few young persons choose medicine solely for selfish gain. Usually, the decision to become a doctor involves a decision to be committed to the good of others, and to helping people who are in need. Unethical doctors are tragic because they usually have fallen from earlier ideals. Between the original self-creating commitment and a final tragic fall, there are many minor failures and bad habits. The original self-creating commitment creates an *ethos* which must be nurtured by repeated good acts in order to qualify as character in the sense of good moral personality. Habitual attitudes joined to their consistent expression in concrete acts are called virtues or vices. Character considerations are closely tied to virtues, and we now turn to look at them.

Notes

1. Kierkegaard, Soren, *Either/Or,* (Garden City, New York: Doubleday), 1959, (2 vol.).

2. Kierkegaard, Soren, *The Present Age,* Alexander Dru, trans., (New York: Harper and Row), 1962, p. 43.

3. Tolstoy, Leo. *The Death of Ivan Illich and Other Stories,* (New York: The New American Library), 1960.

4. Kierkegaard, Soren, *Fear and Trembling and Sickness unto Death,* (Garden City, New York: Doubleday), 1954.

5. Bolt, Robert. *A Man for All Seasons: A Play in Two Parts,* (New York: Random House), 1962.

6. Arendt, Hannah, *Eichmann in Jerusalem: A Report On the Banality of Evil,* (New York: Viking Press), 1963.

7. In the eighteenth century, when pressure was put on physician privilege by free trade advocates, English doctors appealed to character requirements for doctoring. See chapter 14, "Doctors as Priests."

10.

The Ethical Self and the Practice of Virtue

Virtue, like *ethos,* refers to a lived personal dimension of morality. Over the years, however, it has meant different things in different cultures. For the Greeks, *arete* meant lived morality in the sense of noblemindedness. For the Romans, *virtus* signified the same noblemindedness,[1] but with an emphasis on firmness and dependability in private and public life. During the early Middle Ages, virtue as noblemindedness tended to mean chivalrousness. In contact with medieval theology, however, the concept of virtue was expanded to refer to a wider and less militaristic form of lived morality. Today, the term virtue means a disposition toward appropriate acting; what used to be called "habits of the heart."[2] As more or less permanent forms of lived ethics, virtues are closely related to the lived inner reality we have been talking about as *ethos* and character.

Virtue and Other Ethical Categories

Human beings are structurally different from animals in the distance which they enjoy from a reality which emerges for them alone as meaning and possibility. A distance or separateness breaks a unity with the outside, which determines the animals' reactions, but leaves human beings free to respond in varied ways. This human structure is the ground of morality. Not only can persons create their own responses to the outside, they must do so to be themselves. Objective standards for these responses are derived either from some understanding of the universal human structure or from particular bonds like the doctor/patient relationship, and virtues make possible a consistent execution of the standards. Structure, principle, duty, rights, and virtue are major categories of ethics, and all are interrelated.

The lack of perfect correlation among these interrelated categories is explained by the way ethics developed historically. Because ethics is human, it shows the untidiness and richness of any human endeavor over time. Nevertheless, a certain correlativity and order among the basic categories of ethics exist. Principles are rooted in structure and serve as the ground of duties. Rights refer to enforceable claims either for non-interference (negative rights) or for specific acts due to us from others (positive rights). Virtues establish dispositions and habits of living according to objectively right standards.

Sometimes rights talk is more appropriate (when certain behavior must be demanded forcefully). In other contexts, it is more appropriate to speak of principles and duties, or virtue and character, because a different emphasis is required. Usually, for example, it is more appropriate to talk of a Christian duty to charity than of the right to be treated charitably; but with the proper nuances, a case could be made for both expressions. Certainly, it is appropriate to talk of the need to develop the virtue of charity.

Both in the classical tradition and in contemporary philosophy, virtue and character are discussed together. In many cases, the terms are used interchangeably. Chivalry, noblemindedness, dependability, can be understood either as particular virtues or as examples of a person's character. To be considered of good moral character, a person must acquire virtues. Character, however, in the sense of *ethos* or inner ethical being, refers to something less fragmented than particular virtues; a more unified and fundamental orientation of the self.

Virtues and Vision

The interrelation between virtue and character is a subtle one. Efforts at character formation do not produce a fixed thing, and formation does not occur according to a fixed schedule. There are no moral blue prints for becoming an ethical self. Kierkegaard's insistence that ethics begins with an absolute commitment points to the fact that character is not formed the same way a house is built: piece by piece, brick by brick, one discrete action after another, until the project is complete. Rather, for character to be formed, first there must be a radical, creative turning of the self in some definitive direction. Kierkegaard uses the term "absolute commitment" to refer to this move. Before the inner ethical self is forged, there must be a non-conditional commitment of the person to an ideal, a meaning system, a model of existence, or a vision of life. Character precedes virtue in the sense that there must first be a vision of what the desired good is like, and then attitudes and dispositions to follow such a vision.[3]

For the religious believer, making the definitive turn toward a vision of the good is called "conversion," a word which refers to a turning of the whole self toward God in faith. In more secular terms, it could be an unconditional turning of the whole self toward some professional way of life. The good doctor, no less than the good Christian, must first believe that a certain way of life is good, and then throw himself or herself without reserve into the task of realizing it. The unconditional choice or total commitment gives an important first form to character. It serves as the foundation for a further gradual formation through disciplined efforts to acquire the particular virtues characteristic of the chosen vision. Any effort merely to acquire virtues, like piling bricks one upon the other, is obviously an exercise in futility. Deeds repeated one after another lead nowhere and do nothing; but deeds derived from attitudes, informed by a faith and directed toward an ideal can lead to the development of both virtue and character.

In the life of a doctor, no less than in the life of religious believers, virtues can be acquired if the basic vision is kept alive and if effort is expended to conduct one's life in light of concrete models supplied by the vision. It makes as much sense in medicine as it does in religion to make a place for ethics in the sense of personal being, alongside an ethics of rules and principles, and logical arguments. But in neither case, can the effort to acquire virtue be disconnected from an original vision. The vision must be there in the beginning, and it must be preserved in some meaning-giving narrative, and periodically there must be recommitment to the vision's ideals.

Character, initially forged, continues to be formed by virtues as long as the supporting narrative or meaning system is kept alive. Even the Greeks presupposed this dialectic between the inner ethical self and a vision. In Plato's ideal of moral education, for example, there is the vision of the good, which organizes and informs the acquisition of virtues. Keeping an eye on a vision of the good is as important as keeping an eye on one's attitudes and actions and on what is happening to the inner self.[4]

Virtue, then, as lived morality or a lived dimension of morality, refers to a gathering of personal motives, feelings and dispositions for a consistent lived expression of a vision. Virtue is linked with objective moral standards, and expresses objective norms in a personal way. What is distinct about virtue is that the acts in accordance with objective norms or standards come forth from the person without a struggle in every instance over the applications of principles to facts or the calculation of burdens versus benefits. Each new case does not have to be analyzed. Facts and consequences in each new circumstance do not have to be weighed in order to do the good. As lived morality, virtue is a part of the whole life of a person, an energy and an attitude which prevails over obstacles with some ease and responds with just and appropriate behavior as a matter of habit rather than calculation and struggle.

Different virtues are different forms of just and appropriate behavior. Courage, for example, is not the same as justice. And yet there is a relationship among virtues, as the term "cardinal virtues" connotes. Certain virtues form a *cardo* or hinge on which other virtues turn. No virtue is possible without prudence, for example, and prudence itself depends for its development upon justice, temperance, and courage. Courage, like prudence, is linked to many other virtues which could never develop without the strength to endure stress and pressure with grace (Hemingway's definition of courage). Different virtues produce different forms of behavior, and all the basic virtues together create what we call good persons. Ordinarily, good persons respond consistently in appropriate ways without being conscious either of character or the virtue dimension of their behavior.

Sigmund Freud may be understood as one thinker whose theories have undermined traditional and common sense understandings of morality in terms of virtue and character. Freud discovered the roots of morality in childhood and childhood influences. As a matter of fact, however, Freud's ethics was more a confirmation than an undermining of this tradition. Mature morality for Freud means a mature moral agent or character. The key virtues of such a person are truthfulness with oneself and reasonableness regarding the claims of reality.[5] Freud wrote about character,[6] had character, and displayed admirable virtues in his own life. Anyone familiar with his life knows this to be the case. Even people who discredit Freud's ideas about morality cannot help but be impressed by his character and virtues.

Virtue and Character

The term, virtue, refers to something that is real about human life. Not only does virtue facilitate good behavior, but it even colors the way opportunities for moral conduct are perceived. The virtuous doctor, for example, sees the need to spend a few minutes reassuring a frightened patient, whereas someone without developed medical virtues would not even recognize the need. In this sense, it is correct to say that virtue not only orders the inner life of a person but, like character, influences a person's relation to the whole of existence. Virtues enable human beings to discover the moral dimensions of reality, as well as to incorporate moral values into discrete and separate acts.

The concept of virtue, then, is both conceptually and practically close to that of character. Virtues (or vices) structure character. They could be called orientations of character in the sense of balanced, rational patterns of choosing, feeling, and acting in accordance with ideals and standards of goodness communicated by a vision. Virtues are not the whole of ethics, but they contribute to good behavior, good persons, and even to good societies. Virtuous acts contribute both to the good (fulfillment) of others and the good of the acting person by creating a readiness and orientation to right action. As virtue is developed, it provides practitioners with a practical moral wisdom, and with a way of achieving the good which is different from act analysis and norm creation.

Because virtue is an appropriated and lived moral reality, it may appear to be something innate rather than chosen or cultivated. No doubt, certain persons have natural dispositions toward particular forms of good conduct. We all know people who seem naturally kind or naturally orderly, but even these persons need to cultivate their natural dispositions and balance them properly with other innate strengths and weaknesses. A natural disposition may make certain forms of virtue easier for some people, but these same persons need to exercise effort to keep any one virtue from dominating life so as to dry up other forms of moral development.

There are, however, persons not naturally inclined toward a certain type of conduct, but who, nevertheless, learn to be virtuous. After realizing that certain forms of moral conduct are indispensable to good medicine, a doctor can learn to be helpful, kind, caring, respectful, promise-keeping, friendly, and the rest. Understanding the part certain virtues play in a good life is an important first step toward developing virtue. It leads to the development of attitudes or to a change in attitudes. Then comes the discipline, the practice, and the effort to act in certain ways. Eventually, the commendable conduct becomes more natural, and dispositions which were not natural become part of one's "second nature." For this to occur, work and discipline are required. Virtue development always involves effort and always requires prudence to keep moral efforts within bounds. Only when particular virtues (e.g., those required of a physician) are brought into harmony with other more common ones, can one speak of a "good doctor."

Virtues and Vices

But who speaks of virtuous persons these days? Wouldn't it be embarrassing to be called virtuous in this day and age? One of the reasons we hear little talk about virtue is that it tends to sound pious and perhaps self-righteous. Some may even think that virtuous persons infallibly choose the right conduct. Certainly, this is not the case. We already mentioned the inevitable narrowing of perspective entailed in every professional commitment. Correspondingly, virtues associated with such a commitment also have a certain narrowing effect. A doctor committed to serving the health needs of other persons may develop virtues associated with the doctor/patient relationship, but not those associated with other forms of human togetherness. Viewing other persons from the medical mindset limits possibilities for looking at them in other perspectives, and correspondingly limits the good habits or lived ethics associated with other perspectives.

The virtue of medical benevolence, for instance, may distract the practitioner from non-medical forms of the same virtue. Very competent doctors may have nothing to offer a patient once their particular form of beneficence (oncology, psychiatry, surgery) turns out to be useless. The eye specialist, for example, may be morally immobilized before the patient whose eye disease is beyond medical help, despite the fact that such a patient has other serious needs at this point. Many patients today complain about being abandoned by doctors while dying. We have already seen that the development of virtues associated with treatment may leave underdeveloped virtues associated with care. Virtue perfects the human being, but "human perfection" is always far from the perfect.

The development of vices or defects of character, even among good persons, shows us a lot about the human condition. Dietrich Bonhoeffer, who may be one of the saints of the twentieth century, talked about what happened to him and his colleagues after years of resistance to Nazism. His comments illustrate the effects of non-virtuous acts upon character.

We have been the silent witness of evil deeds. Many storms have gone over our heads. We have learned the art of deception and equivocal speech. Experience has made us suspicious of others, and prevented us from being open and frank. Bitter conflicts have made us weary and cynical. Are we still serviceable? It is not the genius that we shall need, not the cynic, not the misanthropist, not the adroit technician, but honest, straightforward men. Will our spiritual resources prove adequate and our candor with ourselves remorseless enough to be able to find our way back again to simplicity and straightforwardness?[7]

Bonhoeffer, in this passage, talks precisely about the effect of habitual deeds upon character. He talks about the development of vices and the difficulty of keeping virtues and character intact. The link between habitual acts and the development of either virtues or vices is here expressed in a straightforward way.

Not everything about virtue, then, is upbeat and positive. Limited virtue can result in thoughtlessness. And a lived quality of conduct can congeal into dull, mechanical habit. In addition, the fact that virtue both amplifies and reduces our very perception of reality's moral dimension, means that it increases responsibility as well as the danger of irresponsibility. Virtue can even degenerate into neurosis in the sense of a compulsion to do the good, or into moral failures, when the rational middle ground between opposite extremes cannot be found. And if the moral effort required for virtue focuses on the self rather than the needs of others, a form of narcissism can result. We have all seen people in love with their own self-righteous selves.

Virtue and the History of Ethics

Despite the limitations and dangers of distortion, virtue is an important, indeed essential, part of ethics. Ethics emerges out of human life, and virtue is lived ethics. The classical systems of ethics differed one from another in that they had different concepts of the good. But all the classical ethical systems centered around virtue. Aristotle's *Nicomachean Ethics* and the second part of St. Thomas' *Summa,* are two of the most important ethics texts in Western philosophy, and both are treatises on virtue. The same is true of almost all ethical systems until Kant.[8]

Immanuel Kant erected an ethics of duty over against the traditional ethics of virtue, which developed into what today is called deontology.[9] Ethics, in this tradition, is concerned with those formal characteristics of acts or propositions which qualify them as ethical and justify their being obligatory. Kant's move from a virtue-based to a duty-based ethics followed from his metaphysics. Virtues are incorporations of goods or duties into a lived reality, and as such, become a "second nature." But, for Kant, communication between "ought" (duty) and "is" (being), or between the realm of freedom and the realm of nature is impossible. Morality as natural or lived morality is split off from rationally grounded duties. Morality, for Kant, remains in the realm of duty and freedom, but not in the realm of nature and virtue. Not even Kant, however, could dispense with the notion of virtue when it came time to develop the empirical dimensions of morality. So virtue in Kant's system becomes the moral willpower to carry out one's duty. Willpower, therefore, applied to different obligations, turns out very much like the notion of virtue in classical tradition which Kant overturned. And no philosopher before or after was more virtuous than Kant in his professional life.

If the complex world of ethics is too broad and too rich to be synthesized within the concept of virtue, the same can be said, with even stronger reason, of the duty concept. Fanatical deontologists who would like to make ethics (including medical ethics) a matter of duties and rational rules, either condemn themselves to inadequacy or slip in under some other name the ethical realities which they set out to exclude. A duty, from the verb *deber*, is what is owed. It connotes something missing, a lack that needs to be filled. Logically, a lack refers to or implies a fullness, and that fullness is precisely what moral philosophers after Kant called values. If one "ought" to do something, it is because what one ought to do "is of value." An ethics of duty logically led to an ethics of value (Hartmann).[10] An ethics of value, in turn, leads right back to the ethics of virtue.

Once the concept of value is forced down from a Platonic world of ideals and pure essences, values become possibilities that are open to appropriation by human beings. Values become inner attitudes, acts, events, which human beings recognize as good and seek to realize. Once appropriated, values become virtues, and the circle is complete. The Kantian system, which turned away from the tradition in which virtue is an essential element in ethics, turns out to be a short-lived deviation. The growing interest in virtue among modern ethicists represents a return to a tradition which is strong and persistent because there is something right about it. Medical ethicists are among the last to make this turn. A purely deontological medical ethics is too formalistic and too abstract. Virtues, on the other hand, represent the concrete, lived dimension of ethics. In the long history of medical ethics before Kant, an ethic of virtues constituted the whole of medical ethics, and the system collapsed under that excess weight. Now after years of neglect, it is time to join medical ethics again with the Western tradition.

Virtue in Medical Ethics

Doctors, like all human beings, are constitutively ethical. In addition, they are publicly committed to helping persons who are in medical need. Each patient and every medical situation provides an opportunity for any number of possible goods (values) to be accomplished. As doctors go through life making value choices and appropriating them into conduct, they constitute themselves as certain types of persons. Certain ethical habits are developed and character is created. Thus, do doctors make a moral life.

We are all condemned to be ethical in the sense of creating our own responses to reality, but we can become good persons only if we work to form habits of good behavior. The standards for this good behavior we bear within ourselves. What we are like as human beings becomes a "law," providing standards and guidelines of right and wrong behavior toward other persons. Because persons are what they are, they must be respected, free, helped when in need, communicated with, educated, and so on. As we have seen, for doctors an added standard of right and wrong is the nature of the doctor/patient relationship. Human beings become good or bad doctors accordingly as they develop those habits required to fill up what is lacking and needed in persons who are ill and come to them for help.

Medical practice, however, changes. Human beings change themselves, and they also change basic human institutions like medicine. But even so, there are certain characteristics we recognize in human beings wherever we find them, and so too, there are enduring characteristics of the helping relationship which is medicine. These become the standards of virtue development. Making right choices, according to standards we find in the structure of human persons and their basic relationships, requires the proper use of reason. Virtue, then, is the personal appropriation of values made with the help of reason. Practical reason, in the sense of deliberation and prudential choice, belongs to the very definition of virtue and is crucial for the practice of good medicine.

Besides this strong intellectual or rational element, virtue also means willpower which Kant emphasized. Impulses and passions are good, but in order to be used effectively in value appropriation, they must be subject to control. The English word "virtue" comes from the Latin *virtus,* which means force or power, and it still retains some of its original meaning. Besides judging what is right, the virtuous person and the good doctor have the power to control their attitudes in order to act according to good judgment.

Conclusion

We can conclude this chapter on virtue by returning to what was said above about its under side. Virtue practiced without a vision of the good, or disconnected from belief about the meaning of life, becomes virtue for its own sake; moral gymnastics or ethical masochism. Certain sectarian forms of western religion showed weakness for just this distortion. Insofar as Kant and later deontologists can be understood as reactions against this tendency, they are right. But as frequently happens, the reaction against one extreme falls into excess at the opposite end.

Ethics generally, but medical ethics in particular, can be strengthened by a return to virtue and character considerations following the deontological corrective. But in order not to fall into past excesses, any virtue talk in modern medical ethics must be firmly rooted in what is peculiar to and characteristic of the work of medicine. After recognizing that there must be a place in medical ethics for character and virtue, we have to ask, "what virtues?" and "what kind of character?" The answer to these practical questions lies in the connection between medical virtues and the doctor/patient relationship in which they are rooted. The first half of this book was concerned with unpacking what is involved in the doctor/patient relationship and showing how the needs of patients constitute the foundations of what a good doctor ought to do and, ultimately, ought to be.

Notes

1. *Aristos* in Greek means noble, and comes from the same root as *areté*, virtue.

2. Bellah, Robert, et. al. *Habits of the Heart: Individualism and Commitment in American Life*, (New York: Harper & Row), 1985. This important book discusses the traditional civil virtues of Americans and the deterioration these have undergone in recent times.

3. This connection between vision and character development has been emphasized and refined by Stanley Hauerwas. See especially, *Character and the Christian Life: A Study in Theological Ethics*. (San Antonio: Trinity University Press), 1985.

4. Plato, *The Republic*, Book VII, 517.

5. Rieff, Philip, *Freud: The Mind of a Moralist*, (New York: Doubleday), 1959.

6. Freud, Sigmund, *Character and Culture*, (New York: Collier), 1963.

7. Bonhoeffer, Dietrich, *Prisoner for God: Letters and Papers from Prison*, (New York: Macmillan), 1958, p. 27. Quoted by Meilaender, Gilbert C. *The Theory and Practice of Virtue*. Notre Dame, IN: University of Notre Dame Press, 1984.

8. Thomas Aquinas, Saint, *Summa Theologica, Second Part of the Second Part*, 1-189. (New York: Benziger Brothers), 1947. Aristotle, *Nicomachean Ethics*, trans. by Sir David Ross, (London: Oxford University Press), 1954.

9. Kant, Immanuel, *Critique of Practical Reason*, (New York: Liberal Arts Press), 1956.

10. Hartmann, Nicolai, *Ethics*, (New York: Macmillan), 1932.

Part III

Philosophical Foundations of an Ethics of Character and Virtue

11.

What the Word "Ethics" Means

Inability to recognize persons (*agnosia*) is considered a disease because seeing and knowing personal features is an essential capacity of human beings. What is true of human beings is also true of the literate philosophical disciplines which strive to understand *good* and *right*. Indeed, recognition of persons and sensitivity to personal development are at the very heart of ethics.

Loss of the personal is tragic in ordinary life, as we saw in the story which opened this book; what is true of life in general is so also in ethics, and doubly so in medical ethics. In order to recover what has been lost, a reconceptualization of the philosophical foundations is required. Without a grounding either in coherent philosophical argument or religious belief, talk about character and virtue may sound nice, but lack substance. Philosophical reasoning about the foundations of ethics draws on subsidary disciplines like etymology, anthropology and sociology. We'll begin with etymology.

The word *ethos* (ηθοσ) is the root of *ethica* (ηθικα) and both terms are important for understanding the meaning of right and wrong. The

Greek word *ethos* referred to the basic orientation or disposition of a person toward life. Originally this word meant an abode or a dwelling place. Later, during the time of Aristotle, it came to mean a person's interior dwelling place. The word was used to refer to what a person carries within himself; his interior attitude, disposition, relationship to himself and to the world around him. *Ethos,* in the sense of a person's very inner being, is the root or font of all particular acts.

This original meaning of *ethos* shows up an aspect of ethics which has been obscured at different times in the long history of ethics. As we have seen, both ethics generally, and contemporary medical ethics emphasize concern with external acts rather than with attitude, disposition, or the inner being of a person. Historically, the word *ethos* was used in the sense of actions, habits, customs, but never exclusively so.

Throughout history, there has been a relationship and indeed, a tension between *ethos,* meaning the inner being of a person, and *ethos* in the sense of habits or customary actions. The word *ethos,* as well as the academic discipline, *ethics,* have emphasized first one and then the other meaning. Medical ethics in our day, however, is so preoccupied with particular actions that the older, original meaning is ignored.

Talk about a person's inner being or the personal root of human actions might be understood biologically: i.e. as that primary and unchosen something with which a person begins life. On the other hand, inner being also refers to that form or character which human beings give their lives or acquire as they act out their personal histories. The etymology of the word "ethics" shows that it originally referred to a person's being in this second sense. *Ethos* was opposed in Greek to *pathos,* i.e., what a person suffers, or what is given by nature. Ethics originally referred to a person's second nature, that inner personal being that is no less real for having been created by human effort. Individual acts contribute to second nature, but ethics is not exhausted by analytic and judgmental considerations of these acts.

The human drama, we could say, is one played out between *pathos* and *ethos,* between what is given and what we do with what we get.

Pathos is not irrelevant. What we start with makes a big difference, but it does not determine our inner being. We can modify our "given," considered either as biology or culture. It is not easy, but the given or first nature can be restructured, and this possibility is both the historical ground and the traditional concern of ethics. Historically, ethics has been occupied with the making of a self or with the constitution of a personality.

Ethics, then, is a drama, but never an act of creation, because the original given—"the old self" or the "first self"—never completely disappears. Human nature, in the sense of that set of capacities and potentialities with which each person starts out, is the raw material of human existence. Human nature is a call to further formation. The "something more" is what each human being does with his primitive given in interaction with other people and the symbols of his culture. Human beings, then, are neither purely natural nor purely ethical creations but a peculiar mixture of both. If we stay too close to the original given, we will be primitive and alienated from our potential. If we choose to become too closely identified with historical or cultural models of the human, we will lose the beauty and spontaneity of "natural" man.

Ethics, as a concern with the inner being which people create themselves, must remain sensitive to the possibility of people making themselves badly. There is no guarantee that the making of a self will be a good work. In fact, just the opposite is a very strong possibility. What human beings decide for their lives can be a distortion. Ethics does not involve only the good. Our very physical given as human animals testifies to this. For example, we blush and feel ashamed. Both behaviors are peculiarly human and totally natural, and both show that nature has its own built-in mechanisms for indicating to us and to others that something is not right.

A person's second nature, or character, or inner being, is formed slowly over the course of life. One person will start out more sensitive, another more open, a third of happier disposition. Sensitivities and sentiments (*pathos*) are the raw materials of our character. We humans can form these, or restrain them, or retrain them, or even distort and destroy them. Customs and institutions, education and professional training play a big role in this process. For example, a major influence on the character of a young doctor is the training received in medical school. It definitely makes sense to talk of a professional personality because doctors are taught to act in certain ways and to avoid certain attitudes; to feel and, at the same time, not to feel. The same is true of priests, nurses, lawyers and other professionals. Because character develops slowly under the influence of many kinds of pressures, it is not always so obvious that inner being is our own creation. What we do with influences and how they combine with our choices to create our second nature, is what the term *ethos* originally referred to and is what ethics originally was all about.

Loss of the original sense of this Greek term was due in part to the Latin language which translated both senses of *ethos* by the one term *mos/moris*, from which we get our words moral and morality.[1] The meaning of *mos* was almost synonymous with *habitus*. The emphasis in Latin was on action—something done, a practice, behavior, conduct. The plural form, *mores*, carried the even more obvious "external" meaning of manners, or customs, or usages. The "internal" sense of *ethos*, as the very being of a person, character, or font of actions, gradually was forced into the background. Ethics or moral philosophy became more and more a science of analyzing and evaluating actions and less and less concerned with a person's inner being.[2]

The English word "moral" is an adjective used to describe something that is considered acceptable. We talk about moral and immoral acts, institutions, and policies. Moral does not refer, as did the Greek term *ethos*, to a person's inner disposition, or interior being. And yet we do have another word, "morale," to describe something very close. We talk of a person's morale being low or high. Such expressions carry a stronger psychological flavor than the original ethical sense, but yet the link between the word "morale" and the lost original meaning of *ethos* can hardly be missed. Morale represents our language's attempt to preserve the notion of an inner place. Ordinarily we would not think of morale as belonging to the field of ethics, and yet etymology points a way to include it as essential. An ethics which retains some consciousness of its tradition as a discipline cannot ignore the morale of the person acting. One hears little about morale in medical ethics literature, but it has a great deal to do with the ethical quality of medical acts.

Ordinary language makes some interesting distinctions between individual acts and the person's inner reality. People speak of so and so as being a good person "down deep"; or a good person despite many not-so-good actions. A "good-natured person" might reveal herself in certain critical life choices and in certain critical acts, rather than in a long series of less important ones. According to common wisdom, a person's *ethos* or character is more important than this or that individual action. This insight, reflected in ordinary language, is true of persons generally, and is especially true of doctors.

But what is this inner dwelling place, or self, or inner being of a person? If it is not given (*pathos*) but made, how is it made? In what sense is a person's *ethos* or character his own creation? What does it mean to talk of a person's inner life as a project from which no one can escape? Do *ethos* and *ethics* belong to a human being's very constitution?

How is a doctor's *ethos* formed? How great an influence on the quality of professional actions is the inner being of the doctor? This essay argues that medical ethics has to be concerned with character; otherwise it is not a complete ethics. For this reason, the next chapter, abstract though it may be, is logically required. The evidence gathered from etymology is not enough. We must continue the philosophical analysis of human being in order to provide a foundation for the relationships between ethics and personal character.

Notes

1. One reason for going back to the Greek in pursuit of original meaning is that the Romans often inadequately translated Greek philosophical terminology, thereby impoverishing much of Greek thought. The Romans were never great metaphysicians and besides, were

at a low point in philosophical creativity when they turned to the task of translating the Greek philosophers.

2. Using philology as a starting point for philosophical reflection is characteristic both of Heidegger and Spanish philosophers like Zubiri and Aranguren. Cf. Aranguren, Jose Luis L., *Etica,* (Madrid: Alianza Editorial), 1983. This section is greatly indebted to this work and to other books by the same author. These books include: Aranguren, Jose Luis L., *Catolicismo, dia tras dia,* (Madrid: Editorial Noguer), 1955; Aranguren, Jose Luis L., *Catolicismo y protestantismo como formas de existencia,* (Madrid: Alianza Editorial), 1980; Aranguran, Jose Luis L., *El buen talante,* (Madrid: Tecnos), 1985; Aranguren, Jose Luis L., *El futuro de la universidad y otras polemicas,* (Madrid: Taurus), 1973; Aranguren, Jose Luis L., *El protestantismo y la moral,* (Madrid: Ediciones Sapientia), 1954; Aranguren, Jose Luis L., *El Quijote y la comunicacion,* (Madrid: Ediciones de Comunicacion), 1983; Aranguren, Jose Luis L., *Erotismo y liberacion de la mujer,* (Madrid: Ariel), 1982; Aranguren, Jose Luis L., *Espana sin ir mas lejos,* (Madrid: Laia), 1982; Aranguren, Jose Luis L., *Espana: una meditacion politica,* (Madrid: Editorial Ariel), 1983; Aranguren, Jose Luis L., *Infancia y sociedad en Espana,* (Madrid: Hesperia), 1983; Aranguren, Jose Luis L., *La comunicacion humana,* (Madrid: Editorial Technos), 1986; Aranguren, Jose Luis L., *La crisis del catolicismo,* (Madrid: Alianza), 1980; Aranguren, Jose Luis L., *La Guerra civil espanola,* (Madrid: Planeta), 1986; Aranguren, Jose Luis L., *La etica de Ortega,* (Madrid: Taurus), 1966; Aranguren, Jose Luis L., *La filosofia de Eugenio d' Ors,* (Madrid: Ediciones y Publicaciones Espanolas), 1945; Aranguren, Jose Luis L., *La funcion social del intelectual,* (Madrid: Editorial Ayuso), 1983; and, Aranguren, Jose Luis L., *Planificacion educativa,* (Madrid: Editorial Nova Terra), 1975.

12.

Ethics' Roots in the Structure of Persons

If someone asks, "what do you do?" and I respond "I teach ethics," or "I write about ethics," a discomfort may immediately be created. "I'd better watch my language around him" or "I'd better be on my best behavior" may be the first thought to cross the other person's mind. Ethics, for most people, is "something like religion" or at least has to do with high ideals. What people tend to think about a professional ethicist they once thought about priests and rulers. A presumption about being a good person, which we still find associated with priesthood, was once equally applied to doctors. In fact, the ethical training of the medieval doctor, as we saw in chapter seven, was the same as that given to the priest.

Ethics and Human Nature

Rather than being primarily a university discipline or the concern of professionals, ethics, in fact, is part and parcel of every human life. Instead of being a system of ideals, far removed from daily life, ethics is a concrete necessity forced upon every person by the very psycho-bio-social structure of human beings. The emergence of human beings from the animal kingdom was indeed an ethical event. It involved the appearance of an ethical being where before there was none. The inescapable ethical dimension of human being becomes manifest in a comparison of animal and human life.

In the animal kingdom, behavior is most understandable within a stimulus-response model.[1] The stimulus or stimulus situation on the one hand and the peculiar biological capacities of the animal on the other constitute a dynamic equilibrium which determines an animal's reaction. There is a built-in adequacy in the animal's behavior. In its basic activities, the animal makes a balanced adjustment, or better perhaps, a balanced adjustment takes place which provides a picture of the animal at one with its world.[2] It is only when animals are ripped out of their natural settings that we see a loss of this adjustment.

The animal, or even more so the insect, witnesses to a harmony between biological capacity and the surrounding stimulus situations. The animal or insect action is adequate to the stimulus situation. It does what is "required" or "demanded" by the situation even when the very life of the insect or animal is at stake (for example, when bees die to protect the hive from a hornet attack, or an animal moves into an inevitably fatal confrontation to protect its young). If we use the one term ad*just*ment to stand for all the evidence of harmony or adequacy in insect and animal behavior, then we can say that there is a certain "*justice*" built into pre-human actions.

The Human Environment

Being animals themselves, human beings inherit some of this built-in equilibrium. Like any other animal, we adjust and adapt to the outside; for example, to small temperature changes and circadian rhythms. Within certain limits, we also adjust to sleep deprivations. In humans, however, there is a greater physiological and psychological complexity than anything we find in the animal kingdom. The human brain is much more highly structured. The environment outside is also more complex, because the human brain permits it to be so variously perceived. Human beings, too, are capable of more complex movements. Their hands, for example, far outstrip the animals' in mobility and corresponding capacities.[3] Human dexterity and external complexity correspond to an internal system we talk about as a person's inner self. All of this together explains why human action, unlike that of the animal, is not an automatic *adjustment*.

Reality is different for each species because their different organisms create different schemes and patterns of reality. And yet with animals, generally, there is an equilibrium between the outside and their particular receptor systems. An animal's reaction is interwoven with what it receives from the outside, which is not the case with us. One could look at a human being as just another animal with a quantitatively greatly enlarged receptor system, but such a view seems inadequate to explain human experience. Human resposes are qualitatively different from animal reactions. Only humans create a culture. Language, art, myth, history, religion, philosophy are only some of the peculiar behaviors which alone belong to the human world.

The human world's unique features are founded on a human bio-psycho-social structure. Because there is no harmonious continuity between a person's bio-psycho-social system and that with which it interacts, human beings are freed from their surroundings.[4] To be a human being means not to be determined in responding to the outside. Because the outside does not dictate a response, human beings must construct a response. The human animal is the only one who does not react directly and immediately.

This concept of humanness as a discontinuity with nature is found in one or another form in the great philosophers of human existence. G.W.F. Hegel's classic analysis of the structure of human consciousness shows that human self-awareness comes to be in opposition with what is set over against it. This separateness of the human from what surrounds him or her has been picked up by other philosophers like Jean-Paul Sartre and Gabriel Marcel. Erich Fromm sees in man's separateness the experience which sacred writers expressed in the symbolic language of man's fall or separation from God. The fall from nature or human separation from the world is, on the one hand, the loss of a built-in adjustment. On the other hand, this break with nature is the beginning of human distinctness. The gap, or fall or break makes it possible for human beings to construct a new set of relationships with the outside. It sets up the condition for the possibility of creating a set of responses which remake the world in man's image. In the process, human beings remake themselves.[5]

The continuity or equilibrium between the outside and inside is broken in the human animal. The "natural" process is interrupted, and a delay between the outside stimulus and the response makes its appearance. This delay, characteristic of the human world, appears to some as a questionable advantage. Comparing the human to other animals, Jean Jacques Rousseau concluded that man was sick. *"L'homme qui medite est un animal deprave."* Others, however, interpret this human phenomenon as a qualitative leap in the evolutionary process. What seems to be an insignificant difference from other animals, perhaps even a weakness, is the foundation both of human freedom and intelligence. That apparently small difference makes possible all of the unique behaviors which set human beings apart as culture makers.[6]

The Natural Roots of Freedom and Intelligence

Freedom begins with delay in the sense of being suspended before a situation. As a result, no action, or reaction, is "naturally" forthcoming. Human beings do so many different things, many times unpredictably, because no one behavior is forced upon them. Because the outside does not dictate a response, human beings have to "take account of" or think about their situation. They must even take themselves into account. The person's very self emerges as a reality which calls for thoughtful response. Humans must consider (from *sidera*—the stars, referring originally to man's observation and reflection on the heavens) a number of different actions that are possible. What we refer to as human intelligence is required by and linked to freedom.

The structure of the animal's sensory apparatus or receptor system pretty well defines what will be a stimulus and what will constitute the animal's environment. To a certain extent the same is true for humans. But, in the latter case, the outside reality is not so well defined. A human person can look at a situation differently, perceive it from any number of perspectives, consider it, conceptualize it, and interpret it according to many different models of understanding. This external lack of specification corresponds to a similar situation within the human person. Both that with which persons respond and that to which they respond is unspecified and undetermined.[7] The human mind permits a move beyond the reality faced into unreality (the situation as a person would like it to be—or how it should be). Human consciousness is, in this sense, transcendent. Given this indeterminacy and lack of specificness, a human action is not necessarily *just*. It is not an automatic ad*just*ment.

Human freedom which has received such high sounding praise from many philosophers has humble beginnings. It is not what Sartre would have us believe—unfounded, uncreated, meaningless. Rather, human freedom, at least in its most primitive form, appears to emerge from a very complex human biology. This same biology founds human intelligence. The human capacity for reasoning, like human freedom, is grounded in man's bio-psycho-social organism. Freedom and intelligence, then, do not remove persons from nature, as Kant and Hegel insisted, but only from the animal kingdom. Freedom and understanding are very much a part of human nature.

Because freedom and intelligence intervene between the outside situation and a response to it, the human response is not given or fixed. Intelligence in man converts what for the animal is a determined environment, into a set of possibilities. Human beings are free from the situation to the extent that they can either respond or refuse to respond.[8] Because of their intelligence, they are able to imagine any number of different responses suggested by a unique perception of the outside. The outside for us humans is not one-dimensional. It emerges as an almost unlimited sea of possibilities. No two human worlds are exactly alike. The possibilities each person faces are different, and the reaction of each person to interpreted possibilities is different. The idea of every person as unique and inhabiting a unique world is awesome and grounds the idea of individual rights.

In the insect, an action is predictable because the reality with which it interacts is one-dimensional or at least very narrow. There is an adequate action prescribed by a harmony between the outside and a receptor system. The action of the insect or the animal is a ad*just*ment. Human beings, on the other hand, must *justify* their actions, because justice does not automatically belong to them. Human beings, then, are ethical in this basic and primitive way, and their being ethical is rooted in their bio-psycho-social constitution. Sartre is right when he says that man is condemned to be free. Another way of talking about this common human experience is to use the term *agent*. Rather than merely being acted upon or reacting, humans experience themselves as actors and as responsible for the justice or injustice of what they do.

It seems clear then, that the requirement of justice or rightness in human acts has to do with their internal structure. Since the human act is not graced with a pre-given harmony, grace must be supplied. Human actions are condemned to be deficient unless an effort is made to supply the quality of justice. A certain degree of adjustment is present by reason of being an animal and sharing somewhat the animal condition. Human structural complexity, however, keeps this harmony and balance from being complete. Nevertheless, human beings do start out with limits within which they must construct their responses. Human behavior is not creation in the sense of a production out of nothing. To say that humans are ethical animals does not mean that they create justice out of nothing. We give an ethical substance to our acts which already have a certain pre-given structure. *Human beings do not create behaviors, but rather give their behavior an ethical quality—a form of justice, rightness, or goodness.*

Justifying Behavior

Justification, which means *to make just*, actually means to give to actions an added form. When we speak of justifying our acts, we mean giving both a form and giving a rational explanation of that form. A human action must be given a shape or form from among the many possibilities presented which are neither pure, nor unlimited. Even with a complex bio-psycho-social structure, reality comes across as offering only certain possibilities. Some of these are more attractive than others. The human structure creates tendencies toward some things and aversions to others. The human person starts out *preferring* some actions and types of response. Before one prefers, there is something brought forward or offered (from the Latin, *ferre, tuli, latus*—to bring). Persons, however, can either follow their preferences or resist them. Justification of human actions, then, means to choose to act in this or that way, to choose this or that form of action, to actualize this or that preference; and then to provide reasons for the choice.

Because human actions are not creations out of nothing, everything about them is not open to justification. Persons are not pure freedom. The bio-psycho-social reality on which the many perceived possibilities are founded, cannot be justified. (An individual finds herself already in a place, and with a language, a culture, a structure, and a history for which she is not responsible). Nor can a person justify those possibilities to which she is naturally more inclined—her preferences. Individuals simply find themselves with certain interests. These are part of what is given; what we can call human *pathos* (in the sense of being suffered or endured). What is not given, however, is the choice from among the possibilities and preferences (the *ethos*). What is to be given or must be given is a particular form of action which is not predetermined. It is in this sense, that human beings are condemned to be ethical.

Justifying the Self

The fact that human beings must make choices and construct actions in one or another way, makes them ethical animals in a primary and fundamental sense. They are, however, ethical in yet another sense. Human actions will be good or bad, accordingly as they are given a good or bad form, or accordingly as they conform or fail to conform to a certain standard. Human beings both choose and choose according to some standard of good and evil. The fact that actions are chosen separates us from animals. In addition, human actions can be chosen not because they conform to an outside reality, but rather because they conform to an ethical standard or because they are made to conform to a certain ideal. In an even more radically ethical sense, the human capacity for choice extends to the very human self, and definitive choice of a certain self made in conformity to some ideal actually creates a self. The inner being, or character of a person, is an ethical creation.

Just as the master craftsman gives an intended form to the things he makes, human beings give a form to the material of human life itself. The making of one's self into a good person: this is the supreme human project. Human beings are ethical both in the sense of making themselves and in the sense of making themselves according to a desired ideal.

Moral theories differ one from another largely in the ideals they recommend or accept as built into the very fiber of human nature (for example, pleasure, power, happiness, love). This is what Aristotle meant when he compared ethical life to what goes on in the technical arts. Humans construct wheels, clothes, houses, cars, societies and finally, somewhat mysteriously, they also construct their own being, and do so with some previous form in mind. Aristotle begins his *Nicomachean Ethics* with the statement, "Every Art and every inquiry and similarly every action and pursuit is thought to aim at some good."[9]

The relationship between ethics and the very structure of the human is deepened when we consider the fact that the human personality or the person's own self is an "object" of his choosing. Authentic religion and good psychotherapy provide persons with realistic insights into themselves and their ways of refashioning or improving the perceived self. Persons have a certain distance even from themselves, such that they can choose one or another self from among the many possibilities presented by culture, religion, or bare intelligence. Not only, then, do they give an ethical form to their actions, but give an ethical form also to themselves. Human beings are radically ethical in the sense that their very selves are a matter of choice, and a choice made according to one or another standard of goodness (a lover, a reliever of suffering, a fulfilled or happy person, a revolutionary, a Christ-like person, etc.). Not without reason does the Greek word, *ethos*, referring to the inner self, develop into *ethics*, which includes a concern for human beings as well as human acts. This dual concern of ethics with actions and character is not arbitrary. Human beings are ethical in the sense of being the source of their ethical behavior and in the sense of being themselves an ethical creation.

Summary

Because the ground just covered is the most abstract and philosophical part of the argument for becoming a good doctor, a short summary of the points covered might be helpful.

1. We have been looking at behavior as an adjustment of action to a situation. In the animal kingdom, this adjustment is pre-given, determined both by the psycho-physical structure of the animal and the limited reality with which it interacts. With the human being, however, there is little pre-given adjustment. Rather, the person has to make the adjustment. Human beings must justify their acts. Their behavior is constitutively ethical in the sense that their response to the reality they confront must be constructed. It would be too much to say that their behavior is created because rather than inventing a response, they choose in every situation from among a number of possible responses. The fact that the possible responses are suggested by the culture or society in which they find themselves gives to ethics a strong social dimension. It is sufficient here to say that the necessity of choosing from among possibilities and preferences makes human beings ethical by the very structure of their being. Parenthetically, it can be mentioned here that medical ethics became the major specialty it is today when science and technology generated preferences and possibilities from which doctors and patients must choose. When there were few possibilities and little doctors could do, medical ethics was more a matter of medical etiquette.

2. The justice or justification which humans are forced to give to their acts is not exhausted by the fact that acts are chosen rather than determined. One type of behavior is chosen over another because it is considered to have a certain justice. An added justification comes from the conformity of an act to a moral standard. Human behavior is more than a chosen adjustment to reality. It is behavior with substantial moral content which comes from being informed by standards of goodness. It is in this sense that St. Thomas, following Aristotle, talks of justice as being virtue itself, rather than an aspect of virtue or just one virtue among others. It is the very nature of human beings to do good in the sense of acting according to some standard of goodness, honesty or justice. Humans, then, are ethical not only by reason of structure but also by reason of content. Their acts have a certain moral substance as well as an ethical form. It remains to be seen how conscience functions in the determination of the moral content of human behavior. Of special interest will be the manner in which doctors form their consciences so as to

give both their medical acts as well as their very professional selves an ethical substance.

3. By looking at the etymology of the words "ethics" and "morals," we saw that these referred originally to the very being of persons and not just to their actions. Our analysis of the human condition also points to the fact that not just human acts but the human being enters into the world of his choice. Given reflective intelligence, the human self becomes something to be rightly perceived and then responded to. Theoretical or reflective reason is the ability of human persons to conceptualize their own existence, and practical reason enables them to distinguish between proper and improper responses in light of ends, goals, ideals and standards. We can, therefore, speak of the human being itself needing to be justified. Not just human acts but the human person can be called just or unjust, moral, immoral, or even amoral.

If, when we speak of the human condition we have in mind man's bio-psycho-social human structure, we can agree with Sartre that he is condemned to be free. Freedom and choice are literally forced upon human beings by the indeterminancy rising out of their internal and external complexity. A multitude of possiblities leaves human beings no alternative but to actualize some and reject others. Lives must be made. We call the way we choose to lead our lives conduct (from the Latin *conducere*—to lead or direct). In this sense every person is ethical, even the most unjust or immoral. Even the immoralist is forced to choose his behavior. We speak of unethical or immoral man only in the sense of ethics as content, i.e., the specific form of life or action, related to a norm or standard. Only in this sense is it logical to talk about immoral man and unethical conduct.

4. The human person, finally, is more than his or her fundamental bio-psycho-social structure. Besides being constitutively free and intelligent, the concrete human being who is forced to make his own responses to surrounding situations is also a being with a personality, a disposition, and a psychosomatic constitution. The person who forms his conduct and his life has certain attitudes and dispositions: energetic or

phlegmatic, optimistic or pessimistic, tired or rested, in good or bad humor. Therefore, all these dimensions of human beings are related to ethics. None is foreign to the ethical enterprise. One does not hear much about fatigue and ethics, or morality and good humor, but this only points up a deficiency in the contemporary ethical enterprise.

Notes

1. Stimulus-response talk does not mean isolated stimuli and one-to-one responses. Gestalt psychologists have corrected this distortion by showing that stimuli do not present themselves separately, but rather, in structured fields. The structuralization is both internal and external, involving both a sensory system and the formalized perceptions with which that system interacts.

2. Tinberg, the Oxford animal biologist, used the phrase "adaptive behavior" which is close to what I am trying to describe by the terms *adequacy* and *adjustment*.

3. The chimp comes close to man in the physical development of the hand. The increased manual dexterity of man might be the result of his increased brain power, more than a particular physical advantage which he has over larger apes.

4. Friedrich Wilhelm Nietzsche refers to the person incapable of resisting reaction to a stimulus as a degenerate. "Only degenerates find radical methods indispensible: weakness of will, or more strictly speaking, the inability not to react to stimuli is, in itself, simply another form of degeneracy." Cf. Friedrich Nietzsche, "Morality as an Enemy of Nature," in *The Twilight of the Idols, The Complete Works of Friedrich Nietzsche,* Vol. 16, (New York: Russell and Russell), 1964.

5. According to religious anthropology, following the break with nature or the world, humans can either move forward and in the image of God remake themselves and the world, or they can regress to some form of animal security. The latter option, however, is always a form of neurosis or psychosis. Given the break, human beings have no choice but to follow in the very footsteps of God. Either humans actualize the freedom and intelligence connected with their break with nature or they refuse their essence and, in effect, choose death. Separateness lifts the human out of physical nature into a new level of being. It is not without reason that this new level is called a higher form. High, in this case, denotes both an evaluative superiority and a danger. It is no wonder that human beings, the apex of evolutionary development, are a danger to themselves and, indeed, to the whole planet.

6. There is a form of "delay" which one notes in the "mysterious" mechanism which triggers bird and fish migrations. Changes in the outside, usually climatic, start up a process within the animal which takes as long as a month to complete. At the end of this "delay," the

migrations begin. This is, however, very different from the type of delay to which we are referring.

7. It may seem that the roving dog is free because of the absence of overt external restraint. The dog is, however, bound even in his roving by the meeting of a fixed external reality with narrowed neurological structures.

8. This is the first level of freedom, called, in scholastic philosophy, *Freedom of Contradiction*, i.e., the freedom to act or not to act. It is distinguished from *Freedom of Specification*, or the freedom to choose specific objects or acts. A third type, called *Freedom of Contrariety*, refers to the freedom to choose good or evil; or to choose in terms of a perceived ethical value.

9. Aristotle, *Nichomachean Ethics*, W.D. Ross, trans., *The Works of Aristotle*, Vol. II, (Oxford: Clarendon Press), 1925.

13.

Persons and Ethics as Essentially Social

Although we spoke about the bio-psycho-social structure of the human person, the focus of the previous chapter was on the biological roots of psychic capabilities. A large brain provides the biological ground for the emergence of a complex reality, and both together serve as the foundation for human understanding and human freedom. Because of the way human beings are biologically structured, individuals have to choose from among different possibilities. Up to this point, it has been the solitary individual who made choices from among different preferences, thereby creating his or her individual moral character. The ethical task as we have thus far described it, falls squarely on the shoulders of the individual human actor.

Ethics is actually an individual or solitary project in many ways. We human beings make our lives according to models of life which attract us and influence us. Different models of life, styles of behavior, or ways of being pass before the tribunal of an individual's conscience before one or another is decided upon. "I'll be a doctor" or "I'll be like my father" or "I will make a military career" or "I'll study biology because I admire Dr. Gracia, my biology teacher" or "I'll make every effort to pattern my life on Jesus Christ or Isaiah." Only the individual makes the crucial life creating and character forming decisions, and afterward, the thousands of smaller choices required to incorporate a chosen model into the fabric of a life. The virtues and habits which we have discussed are linked to concrete models in an individual's life. So, the big life choices and little acts required to realize them, a sense of responsibility for one's life and the cultivation of appropriate professional habits, all these ethical realities primarily concern the individual person.

And yet, the individual obviously is immersed in a tangle of relationships. To look at ethics in terms of solitary beings making decisions about their own lives is to do violence to the human reality. Human beings are brought up in social groups, beginning with the family, stretching into all sorts of intermediate institutions (e.g., churches), and to the dominant social patterns of a particular culture. There are solitary individualistic dimensions of life but human life is not reducible to them. The patterns or processes of interrelationship are also a part of life and therefore, part of ethics.

What individuals do with their lives then, is influenced by others and inevitably affects other people. What people choose to be is influenced by close ties with others and works for the advantage or disadvantage of themselves and others. In making themselves, persons are not just influenced by patterns of relationships, but contribute to patterns which influence others. The human person is inserted into a broader social reality, and loyalty to one's group figures historically as a fundamental ethical value. Human solidarity with other persons gives to individual ethical choice and behavior a transpersonal or social dimension. This is true of ethics in general, but especially true of medical ethics.

The Social in Traditional Medical Ethics

From the Hippocratic era until our own, doctors were expected to learn to be good by immersing themselves in a medical society and imitating the example of models provided by their teachers. How did the young doctor learn the ethical skills required of the practicing physician? He watched the way his teachers behaved and imitated their example. Medicine has changed in many ways over the 2,500 years since the beginnings of the Hippocratic tradition, but the system for transmitting ethical formation to the developing physician has remained fairly constant. During the last decade, most medical schools added courses in ethics to the curriculum, but before that time, medical ethics was understood in terms of character traits and taught in relationship with other doctors.

Both within medicine and outside, ideals and models of behavior are important because they become "norms" for others. Finding myself in an unforeseen and unforeseeable situation, I could invent out of the blue the adequate response and (if both situation and response can be generalized) create thereby a new norm or model which might come to constitute an addition to humankind's moral storehouse. If I happen to be a great moral reformer, it is even possible that I invent a new way of life; a new model of human existence. All this is possible but not probable. Most people are limited to choosing in a more or less personal manner, from already established possibilities. These possibilities change and so do social patterns and styles within professions. For example, today we see yuppies with their distinctive ethical styles and yuppie doctors. The Victorian, on the other hand, is a model which has almost completely disappeared. Older doctors set an ethical standard characterized by personal attention both to patient and family. We see this changing today with the emergence of specialists focused on the patient alone. These social changes influence how individuals choose. If we were to require that each individual invent in every case his or her own response, we would be forced to assume that each person stands as an isolated ethical genius. "Authenticity," in such an understanding, would prohibit the moral agent from learning anything from others.

The real human person is different. Human action does not occur in a vacuum. What people do with their lives, they do in a social context. In the great majority of situations, the individual already has the "pieces," or elements, of a moral response furnished either by close family ties or by intermediate groups like churches, or by a particular society, and these pieces are internalized as intrapsychic structures. In many cases, the individual is supplied not only with the different pieces out of which he or she constructs a response, but the whole model of behavior might already be constructed and tailor-made to the circumstance. Patterns of interdependent relations provide moral agents with pieces of practical wisdom, along with overall models of how to act. What is true of society in general is even more true of the smaller, professional societies.

The Social Dimension of Ethics

To say that human beings are socio-culturally determined in their conduct is too strong. We talked about individuals making themselves, and rightly so. But it is equally correct to say that human beings are made by their interdependent relations and the cultural-historical-professional world to which they belong. Human beings create their own worlds, and at the same time the world is already made for them in the sense that they are born into a family, a language, a religious group, an economic-political order; and each of these groups will supply models and norms of conduct. The action of groups upon us is both positive and negative. The social dimensions of life both open up a path before us and confine us to a path. It may be a generalization, but not untrue, to speak of persons developing militaristic attitudes from being raised in a military family and attending a military school. The same type of social influence on character development, we see in medicine. Civilized societies, then, can be said to form their members, but not to the extent insisted upon by orthodox Marxists. It is one thing to insist on the role of society in moral behavior; another to hold that "it is not the consciousness of men that determines their existence, but their social existence that determines their consciousness."[1]

Disavowing this Marxist exaggeration, one can, nevertheless, affirm: 1) that from the point of view of lived morality, moral individualism is certainly not historically primary, 2) once an individualistic morality makes its appearance, it continues to be conditioned by the individual's group associations. We see evidence of this in class and group prejudice where attitudes toward other persons, along with set patterns of behavior toward them, derive from the group. The same influence is also evident in group interests which manage to camouflage themselves as moral norms: e.g., "Patients should obey their doctor's orders," or, "Government should not interfere with the freedom of doctors to practice medicine." The moral conditioning of groups is evident, too, in the economic and intellectual possibilities which they provide for better situated persons and deny to the socially less fortunate. The economic and intellectual opportunities of the upper classes go along with moral opportunities, which are denied to the economically deprived.

Not only does society supply individuals with moral paradigms, attitudes, and opportunities, but individual moral conscience only gradually evolved from a dominant social morality. From the point of view of a psychology of morality, the individual conscience is a late-comer in the history of lived morality, and today's psychological and moral individualism is more a distortion than an evolutionary advance. Psychogenetically, the tribunal of conscience is the interiorization of the community's tribunal. Judgment took place before the *polis,* or on the battlefield, or in the theater, and usually through the application of precepts originating in a religious community. A full-blown morality of conscience was preceded by a group morality. This social reality gets little or no support today either from the mass media which promotes "what feels good or is best for me," or from American schools which ignore public moral education entirely.

History does not count for the individualist; neither does society, nor the needs of community. The only moral standard is that which promotes one's own personal wishes or fulfills one's particular needs. Personal well-being is the guiding ethical principle, and it affects doctors as it does all of us. But doctors today are exposed to harsh criticism because they act like everyone else, looking out for their own selfish interests first. An exaggerated individualism is never attractive, but when doctors come over as interested in "#1" first, they turn out to be particularly disappointing. People expect doctors to operate according to different standards.

Social Ethics or Ethics of Conscience

Ethics, in the sense of a morality of conscience is not necessarily synonymous with an exaggerated individualism. It depends upon the development of an individualized internal forum, but it may involve concern for others and for the needs of community. Usually a morality of individual conscience develops at a time of cultural crisis when the accepted social morality shows itself to be inadequate, ineffective, and unjust. Faced with such a situation, persons retreat into themselves. They take refuge in the intimacy of their moral conscience in order to preserve their integrity. In the example of Socrates, we see an instance of the antithesis between social or group morality and an individual internal forum, as well as the drama associated with this public-private split. When faced with a conflict between what was right according to societal standards and his own personal convictions, Socrates did not duck the punch with a move toward moral individualism. He would not deny the validity of the social norms or even escape their sanction. Yet, in the internal or individual forum, he maintained his innocence. Socrates assumed the stance of an observer of the pull of both the group and the individual person, without deciding in favor of one or the other. The Stoics, whom Socrates criticized, moved closer to an exclusively individual morality, but it was not until modern times that a full-fledged moral individualism showed itself.

An important step toward individualism was taken during the Middle Ages, with changes in the practices of confessors and spiritual directors. Individualistic solutions were forged with the help of a well-developed ethical system called casuistry. The morality of the Middle Ages was social, with norms learned in the family which derived from the church and particularly from monastic communities. As life became more secular, the other-worldly group morality required more and more adaptation. Lacking a grand scheme of any kind to take the place of the traditional social system, the adaptation was carried out case by case. No one dared openly criticize the public moral code (for fear of the Inquisition). At the same time no one knew quite what to do about it. What actually took place was a gradual slip from the plane of a homogeneous social or group morality (which had become more and more problematic) toward the plane of the individual conscience. The question of whether or not a certain act was objectively right or wrong gave way to more modest formulations: "To what degree was so and so guilty when he did this or that?"

We see something of the same type slide in modern medical ethics. Many doctors refuse to work for the development of objective ethical standards valid for the whole society, or even for their own institutions, but insist rather on societal trust as they make their own individual decisions depending on the circumstances of each particular case. Medieval casuists at least worked with standards and norms derived from paradigm cases and widely held principles, but recalcitrant situationist physicians refuse standards of any kind. Following an acceptable procedure or method is as close as they will come to objectivity.

By the eighteenth century, the inherited crisis of the official public morality had gone far enough to permit Kant to formulate his individualistic ethic, attentive exclusively to the internal tribunal of the moral conscience. A transition to the internal forum was now complete, and moral individualism formally inaugurated. This development, however, was followed immediately by reactions of utilitarianism on the one hand and left wing Hegelianism on the other. The period of moral individualism actually was no more than a brief parenthesis in the history of ethics, which was predominately a history of social or group morality.

Ethics in the sense of the philosophical reflection upon morality (a philosophy of morals) developed historically as a secularization of religious morality. The Judeo-Christian tradition has an objective moral system formulated in terms of persons defined first and essentially, as members of a community. From four through ten, the Commandments are an expression not of an individual, but of a group morality. Right and wrong are determined on the basis of an action's influence on the community. During the Middle Ages, a rational or philosophical ethics called Natural Law Ethics, provided a secular foundation for the social norms previously grounded only on religious belief. What was presented in religion as commandment of God, Natural Law Theory spoke of as built into the very nature of human persons and discoverable by the use of reason. Kant makes the next major move with his affirmation that human beings do not discover the laws in themselves but rather give themselves the laws. In Kant's position the movement from external, objective (social) to internal, subjective (individual) morality comes to an end. Right and wrong, which earlier was a judgment founded upon objective social values, now becomes a subjective judgment made by each individual on the basis of what he or she judges to be right or wrong. The judge and the judgment become merged into a single subject who is both independent of other persons and isolated from community. Morality becomes a question of personal merit, dependent upon the good will or proper intention of socially isolated, free individuals.[3]

The Essential Sociality of Ethics

Kant's capital sin was to ignore the fact that human beings are locked in interrelationships, and human action takes place within communities. What a person does has social antecedents and inevitably will have social consequences. We are inextricably bound up with others. We form our own characters in interdependent relationships with others and what we make of ourselves contributes to what others will become. Rather than being an exclusively individualistic project, ethics is carried out in solidarity with one's fellows and in responsibility of each for each. For doctors to think that an ethical medical practice is a strictly private affair between themselves and patients is to ignore the structure of persons, the history of ethics, and especially, the long history of medical morality. But American doctors are influenced by American cultural patterns, and consequently, they mount considerable resistance to public standards, even when these originate in the Council on Ethical and Judicial Affairs of the American Medical Association.

Kant's ethics of good intention, which Weber called *Gesinnungsethik,* continues to influence American ideas about morality. Utilitarianism was a reaction against Kant in the direction of recovering a social dimension to moral thought. Weber placed subjective *Gesinnungsethik* at one extreme and on the other he located an ethic of cynical moral opportunism, attentive only to quantifiable result, which he called *Erfolgesethik.* Between the two is *Verantwortungsethik*—an ethic of responsibility or *Wirklichkeitsethik*—a reality ethic. One need not follow Weber's categories, but it is hard to argue with his insistence upon a socio-cultural dimension of ethics.

Ethics has to be dragged out of its subjectivistic and individualistic confinement by the recovery of its social dimension. Back in touch with Western tradition, questions of right and wrong can be raised in society generally and especially within smaller groups like the hospital or medical society. Many moral philosophers today are aware of the necessity of striving for something more than purity of intention, or a linguistic analysis of formal ethical propositions. Objective moral standards, in the sense of group standards, are sought after by ethicists working in public policy. This is not to say that intention and good will, virtues and character, are irrelevant. Group standards cannot be implemented over the will of individuals. The important thing is to insist that ethics does not stop with interior disposition or the autonomous choice of a single individual. An ethics which points toward making society or a profession, or a particular institution, objectively better does so, not against an individual, but at the same time not contingent upon each individual deciding for himself what is right and wrong.

There is nothing novel about this notion of ethics as social in the sense of being based on the reality of human interdependency or of medical ethics which takes seriously character developed in human relationships. It is hardly more than an application of a traditional concept of "subalternation" to ethics. A subaltern is something of inferior rank serving a higher reality. It is usually used in logic to refer to propositions of inferior rank (particular) serving higher ones (universal), but it refers as well to an auxilliary science serving a superior one. Traditionally, psychology was considered in this relationship to ethics, especially where there was concern with limits of awareness, attentiveness, or mitigating emotional circumstances (sufficient reflection, full consent of the will). Ethics, however, cannot be limited to psychology. Biology, psychology and sociology are all important for ethics.[4]

The intention of this turn in ethics toward the real in the sense of social interdependency on the group is not equivalent to reduction of ethics to sociology. Directing attention to the social does not imply that ethics is nothing more than group conditioning. Even if a person literally accepted every judgment provided by his group, or fulfilled in minute detail everything a medical code required, the autonomous personal moment would still not be eliminated, neither would the issues of virtue and character. In such a case, relationships and society would supply models of conduct ready-made and complete in every detail. This, however, is as unrealistic as the creative individual response in every situation. What we need is a more realistic alternative to our present system in which each doctor alone determines what is right by responding in the privacy of his own conscience to each new situation, and without concern for character and habits of behavior.

Conclusion

This final chapter points not to a moralization of sociology but rather to the social dimension of ethics and especially, medical ethics. A philosophical analysis of the human condition shows human beings to be constitutionally free, and thereby forced to make their behavior just. Just as surely as individual human persons are forced to choose and to be ethical, they are also forced to live in a socio-cultural reality which is also ethical. It comes forth from human beings and incorporates human values. It also turns back on human beings in the sense that it substantially conditions their value decisions. Ethics, in so far as it is human, must be both radically personal and radically social, both private and public. What is true of ethics generally is especially and particularly true of medical ethics.

This emphasis on the social is a necessary corrective to an individualistic American medical ethics. Patients and doctors are frequently understood as if they were disembodied free agents. Consequently, medical ethics is thought of as a negotiation between individuals structured so as not to infringe on, or diminish the autonomy of either agent. Paternalism becomes a major concern in such a view, because it threatens a patient's free choices. One gets the impression from looking at the American medical ethics literature that informed consent is everything.

William F. May, in his book, *The Physician's Covenant,*[5] moves medical ethics in the direction of broader social considerations and intermediary groups. Renee Fox for years has argued that more attention must be paid to social factors influencing moral choices in medicine, and has also called for a medical ethics which makes a place for conditioned habits (virtues) appropriate to doctors who are social beings. "The restricted definition of 'persons as individuals' and of 'persons as relations' that pervades bio-ethics makes it difficult to introduce and find an appropriate place for values like decency, kindness, empathy, caring, devotion, service, generosity, altruism, sacrifice and love. All these involve recognizing and responding to intimate and non-intimate others in a self-transcending way."[6]

Both Alasdair McIntyre, in his book *After Virtue*,[7] and Philippa Foot, in *Virtues and Vices*,[8] have given support to a move toward an ethic of virtue and character. Both authors have called attention to the inadequacy and essential incompleteness of rule dominated ethics, whether derived from utilitarian or Kantian suppositions.

But conclusion of this essay should be characterized as *both/and* rather than *either/or*. For doctors should also pay attention to their tradition, with its emphasis on individual virtues and character. The realities of character and habits of the heart are important to becoming a good doctor. And so, too, are commitments to solving public medical issues and public policies for helping the needy get adequate medical care. The medical tradition includes public commitment and objective norms as well as character development and medical virtues. If doctors do not pay attention to their tradition, which moves in both of these directions, they will become more and more like the rest of us in American culture: preoccupied with facades rather than substance. The phony or selfish doctor, however, turns out being uglier than the similarly distorted lawyer, politician or businessman: more repulsive, more offensive, and more of a scandal. Maybe this tells us something about what makes a doctor different.

Notes

1. Marx, Karl. *The Contribution to Critique of Political Economy*, S.W. Ryazanskaya, trans., Maurice Doll, ed., (London: Lawrence and Wishart), 1971. First published in 1851. p. 20, 1.

2. A morality of honor is one example of a former social medical ethics. It can be seen in many literary works of the Golden Age. A particularly good example for our purposes is *El Medico de Su Honra*, by Calderon de la Barca.

3. Presupposed in this last formulation is a secularized Pelagianism typical of eighteenth century thought (man is essentially good). This is difficult to take seriously after Auschwitz,

Dachau, My Lai, and the violence-ridden life of Central and South America, as well as of our own country's urban centers.

4. Political economics, it may be said, is a special case. Certainly we have in economics a case of subalternation in the above-mentioned sense. At the same time, however, since economic decisions are all human, they have a morality all their own: a morality of special gravity, one might add, because of the link between the decisions of political economics and the lives of so many people. From the eighteenth century on, the most influential moralists in Western culture have been economists: Adam Smith, Bentham, Mill, and Marx, to mention only a few.

5. May, William F., *The Physician's Covenant,* (Philadelphia: Westminster Press), 1983.

6. Fox, Renee C. and Judith Swazey, "Medical Morality is Not Bio-ethics: Medical Ethics in China and the United States," *Perspectives in Biology and Medicine,* Spring, 1984.

7. McIntyre, Alasdair. *After Virtue,* (Notre Dame, IN: Notre Dame University Press), 1981.

8. Foot, Phillipa, *Virtues and Vices and Other Essays in Moral Philosophy,* (Bentley: University of California Press), 1978.

Index